Pilates Workout

LYNNE ROBINSON

and **GERRY CONVY**

FRIEDMAN/FAIRFAX
PUBLISHERS

A FRIEDMAN/FAIRFAX BOOK
Friedman/Fairfax Publishers

Please visit our website: www.metrobooks.com

2002 by Michael Friedman Publishing Group, Inc.

First published in Great Britian 2000 by Pan Books an imprint of Pan Macmillan. This edition published by Friedman/Fairfax by arrangment with Pan Macmillan.

ISBN 1-58663-531-X

1 3 5 7 9 10 8 6 4 2

Distributed by Sterling Publishing Company, Inc.
387 Park Avenue South
New York, NY 10016
Distributed in Canada by Sterling Publishing
Canadian Manda Group
One Atlantic Avenue, Suite 105
Toronto, Ontario, Canada M6K 3E7
Distributed in Australia by
Capricorn LInk (Australia) Pty Ltd.
P.O. Box 704
Windsor, NSW 2756, Australia

Contents

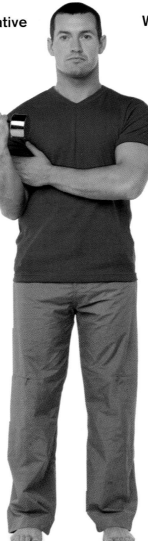

Acknowledgements

Writing this book has been a real learning curve for me. I was leaving my safe haven of Pilates and entering the whole new world of 'gym culture' It has been something of a cross fertilisation experiment! I was fortunate enough to have five men to guide me and act as my mentors. Gerry, my co-author was extremely patient in helping me to understand the equipment and the terminology behind gym and aerobic training. I also want to thank Bryn Kennard, for both reading the script and coming up with excellent suggestions – he has been a wonderful source of information and enthusiasm! Paul Massey, our consulting physiotherapist, gave us sound advice from the medical angle, so we could be sure that our technique was safe, effective and totally in line with the latest research. Man number four, Jeremy Topham-Smith kindly agreed to be photographed and, at the same time, lend us his personal training experience. And last but by no means least I must thank my main man – Leigh, who for some strange reason continues to put up with me, can't think why!

Lynne

Gerry and I would both like to thank everyone at Macmillan for helping us to put this book together. Special thanks to Raymond Turvey, the illustrator who interpreted our ideas and put them down on paper as wonderful illustrations.

There are many people who have helped us directly with this book and I would like to echo Lynne's thanks to them in her acknowledgements. I would also like to pay my respects to just some of those who have personally aided me in my growth as a human being and as a professional.

First of all I would like to thank Lynne for all her help and for giving me the opportunity to express just some of my thoughts onto the pages of this book. Rob Lock is my inspirational Martial Arts coach and great friend. Rob's huge personality, energy, hunger for knowledge, humour and humility are a constant inspiration to me. I would also like to thank Anne Baddeley whose belief in me has recently helped take me to another level in my career. Anne, like Rob has positive energy and personality in abundance and gives me a great lift every time I talk to her. Neil Geraghty is a superb Pilates teacher who has given me a great deal of help during the last three years.

I currently have and have had in the past some wonderful clients and I thank them all for allowing me to help them achieve their goals. I would especially like to thank the Stewart family who have shown me endless kindness throughout my time with them so far.

My own family have given me the platform to express myself, to be unafraid of taking risks, live for the day and still be a good person.

My biggest thanks must go to my beautiful wife Emily who continues to give me endless encouragement, support and love and the freedom to chase my dreams and ambitions. She is the one of the strongest women I know and I appreciate the sacrifices she makes for me.

I have many friends who I must thank for their friendship alone. I would like to think they know who they are.

Gerry

Foreword

Pilates has grown in popularity in recent times due particularly to a new approach to teaching and to a major improvement in the availability of classes. This is due in no small measure to the work of Lynne Robinson and the Body Control Pilates team in building awareness for the Method and establishing new teacher training programmes.

Pilates is a conditioning method that enhances the action of the correct muscle systems. It is safe, enjoyable and effective.

There has also been a boom in the numbers of people who regularly visit health and fitness clubs, where they are confronted by a wide variety of equipment for aerobic and resistance exercise. The correct use and application of this equipment is critical in order to avoid injuries. Incorrect use or inappropriate methods leads to problems (whether through misuse, overuse or abuse), which, in turn, leads to injury.

PILATES WORKOUT is a significant step forward in ensuring the correct use of specific gym-based equipment by applying proven Pilates principles. This means safe exercising in the gym and a reduction in potential injuries. As a physiotherapist who works with élite athletes, I know how important this is.

Lynne and Gerry have combined the worlds of Pilates and gym work in a comprehensive way that you will find both enjoyable and beneficial.

Have Fun!

Paul Massey BA MCSP SRP
Chartered Physiotherapist.

Physiotherapist at the Olympic Games 1992, 1996, 2000.

Physiotherapist to the Great Britain Swimming Team and Great Britain Athletics Team.

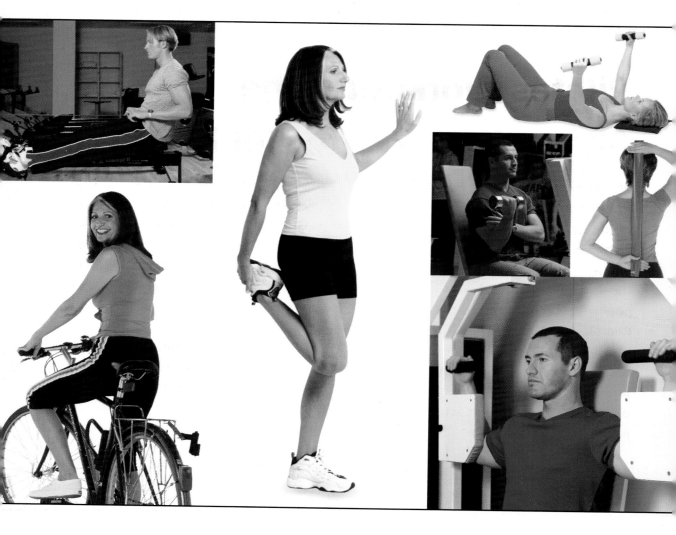

Pilates Workout – The Alternative Way to Get Fit

We have never had it so good with regard to today's 'get fit' options. Enter any sports centre or health club and you are faced with a dazzling array of choices. Body Pump™, kick boxing, aerobics, weight training, spinning and the increasingly popular mind-body techniques including Pilates, tai chi and yoga. But does one method hold all the answers? We don't think so, we all need a mix of activities to provide the perfect balance between flexibility and strength, stamina, speed, skill and cardiovascular health.

What we need above all, however, is to learn how to exercise and move correctly.

This book will show you how to workout safely and effectively both at your local gym and at home, incorporating all the principles of the Pilates Method with its emphasis on safety and good movement. You will be amazed at how subtle alterations to your exercise technique will provide profound and lasting results.

It's true that, 'It's not what you do, but the way you do it'. By changing the way you exercise, you will change the way you look and feel.

The Aim of This Book

Our aim is to introduce you to an alternative way of exercising. What really counts with all these activities is that you use your body correctly as you move and that you have good alignment and sound muscle recruitment patterns. That's what this book is all about: correct body use while you exercise, whether it be on the treadmill, the bike or the rowing machine, or whether you are stretching or lifting weights.

The dangers of poor posture and 'thoughtless' exercise in a gym are evident.

We should be aware of what our whole body is doing while we are performing an exercise. For example, let's take the 'Lat Pull Down' exercise that is commonly performed in many gyms. Are people aware that they are pushing through the balls of their feet as they pull the weight down? Do they realise that they are working out of alignment and therefore risking injury to their lower back? Are they breathing correctly? These are just three examples of body awareness and technique that apply to this particular exercise. Many more are described later on in this book.

What people do not realise is that not only are they wasting their time when they workout incorrectly because the right muscles are not being used, but they also risk injury and long-term damage. We are going to show you the right way to exercise. Not only will this increase the effectiveness of your workout, but it will help to keep you injury free.

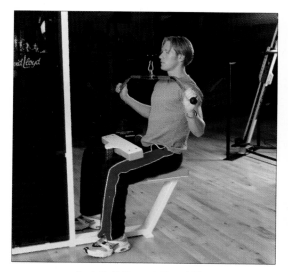

'Lat Pull Down' Good Use

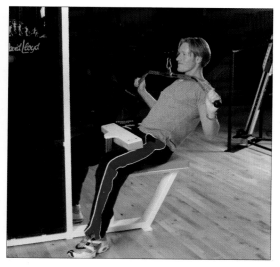

'Lat Pull Down' Bad Use

In the Gym or at Home

Once we have explained the different 'ingredients' of our balanced programme and why they are important, we will introduce you to the Six Golden Rules which you need to understand before you start the workouts. Don't skip these as they are pivotal to the success of the whole programme.

Once you have taken the Six Rules on board, you can either follow the programme at your local gym or at home. Use this programme for eight weeks, then, if you wish, you may take a complete week off – but no longer. You can keep the body supple by doing those Pilates exercises which do not use weights, and by adding gentle stretches. You will not lose anything by resting. In fact, when you resume training you will feel mentally and physically refreshed and the quality of your workouts will continue to improve.

This should be a continual practice during any fitness programme.

We advise you to keep a journal or diary, recording your workouts and your mental and physical reactions, to monitor what is working for you and what is not (see page 112).

Remember to be patient in developing your technique. We are providing you with a solid base to work from, but where you progress to from here is totally dependent on your future goals. Achieving your goals doesn't just start and end in the gym or at home, but in every aspect of your lives. Becoming more aware of how we stand, sit and move will make working out in the gym easier and more effective. Start getting to know your body.

Quality takes time, but it is worth the wait.

The Right Ingredients

Our fitness programme will include the following types of exercise:

Establishing Sound Movement Patterns	↻
Joint Mobility	🚴
Flexibility	🤸
Strength Work	🏋
Aerobic Work	♡

Establishing Sound Movement Patterns ↻

Let's take a brief look at how movement takes place. Starting with the basic frame, the skeleton.

Bones go nowhere by themselves, they need muscles to move them, so we can now add the muscles.

The Skeletal Frame
(main bones and joints indicated)

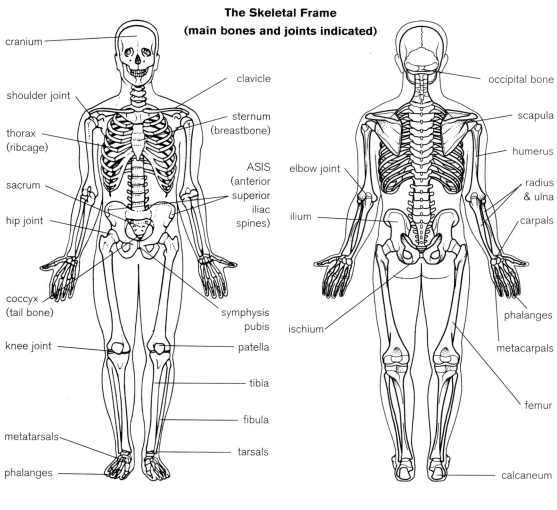

cranium

clavicle

shoulder joint

sternum
(breastbone)

thorax
(ribcage)

ASIS
(anterior
superior
iliac
spines)

sacrum

hip joint

coccyx
(tail bone)

symphysis
pubis

knee joint

patella

tibia

fibula

metatarsals

tarsals

phalanges

occipital bone

scapula

humerus

elbow joint

radius
& ulna

ilium

carpals

ischium

phalanges

metacarpals

femur

calcaneum

Front

Back

You have three types of muscle: smooth, cardiac and striped:

* Smooth muscle is to be found mainly in the viscera.
* Cardiac muscle is the heart muscle and we will, of course, be working on cardiovascular strength in our workout (see page 53).
* Striped or skeletal muscle is arranged in bundles, usually parallel to each other, and this is the muscle we are concerned with in our main programme.

The Muscles
(main superficial muscles indicated)

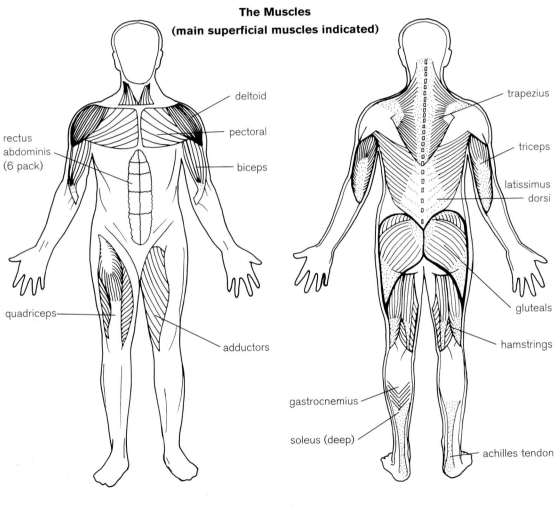

deltoid

pectoral

rectus abdominis (6 pack)

biceps

quadriceps

adductors

Front

trapezius

triceps

latissimus dorsi

gluteals

hamstrings

gastrocnemius

soleus (deep)

achilles tendon

Back

But there's much more to movement than bones and muscles. We also have to consider the 'control', the 'intelligent' part of the system – the nervous system.

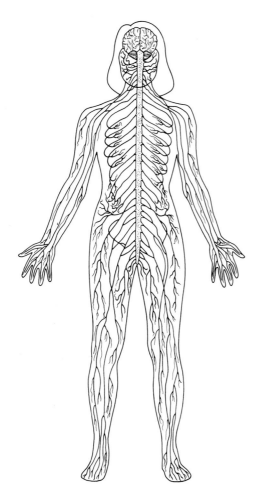

Pathways of the nervous system

There are, therefore, three parts to your body's movement:

1. Nervous system: message, control
2. Skeletal structure: bones, joints, ligaments, cartilage, passive
3. Musculature: active

Muscle is controlled by the nervous system which sends electrochemical energy impulses from the brain, signalling the muscle fibres to contract which makes the bones move. Muscles can only pull (contract), they never push. As they contract the muscle fibres shorten and the opposing muscle must pay out and lengthen for movement to take place efficiently. Muscles are attached to each end of the bone by tendons; the end that stays still is called the origin or proximal attachment; the end which pulls and moves, the insertion or distal attachment.

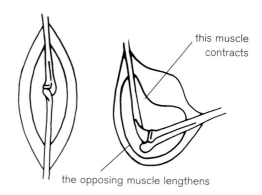

this muscle contracts

the opposing muscle lengthens

For a muscle to contract effectively, the opposing muscle must be able to lengthen and release

You can see from this that movement depends on constant input and output of messages to and from the control room of the brain which remembers patterns, or sequences, of movement, rather than individual muscle contractions. What is now starting to come to the fore in medical research is the importance of good input. What you put into your body in terms of movement is what you get out of it: put in bad movement and you will pick up bad movement patterns, but if you repeat good movement sequences enough times through good exercise correctly executed they become muscle memories and are locked into the brain's muscle memory banks.

This has an amazing effect on how you move and you will not only achieve your goals as far as a great-looking body is concerned, but you will also ensure that your body moves normally. This means less injury and fewer problems.

Joseph Pilates recognised this when he repeated his favourite quote from Schiller: 'It is the mind itself which builds the body.'

Muscle, therefore, is dependent upon and reflects not just individual movements but patterns of use, both good, bad and absent! Lack of use and/or misuse will have an effect on muscle function. Unfortunately, most of us both misuse and disuse our bodies. We no longer perform the wide range of activities for which our bodies were originally designed – running, skipping, jumping, climbing and so on. Instead, we spend far too much time sitting, and sitting badly for that matter, and our activities tend to be repetitive day in day out. This affects both the length and strength of our muscles and their functions, and may ultimately bring the body out of good postural alignment.

Compare the two figures left. Notice where the plumb line falls with Figure A, and note how, with Figure B, many of the bones have shifted forward or back away from the mid line. The joints are no longer in their natural 'neutral' positions, which will affect how gravity falls through the joints. As a result, these may be subjected to increased wear and tear (see pages 10–11).

One of our primary goals in this programme is to help you to find your correct postural alignment – in particular, your natural neutral pelvic and spinal positions – and then to relearn and re-educate the body in how to move well. Getting to know your body doesn't just mean getting to know your postural type. Think about old injuries where you get aches and pains and the effect these have on your body. We can only give you a general overview, but educating yourself will help to accelerate the rate at which you achieve longer-lasting results. Until you have this right, any work you do in the gym will only serve to reinforce bad movement patterns. We have to get it right from the start!

The Girdle of Strength

The importance of the stabilising muscles is becoming increasingly clear in medical research. Let's say for a moment that you want to reach up to take a book from a high shelf. Which muscles do you think would be the first to engage? The hand or shoulder muscles perhaps? The answer is the deep postural muscles, those that support the spine. It makes sense. You don't want to fall over while you reach up. These deep muscles are the ones that stabilise the

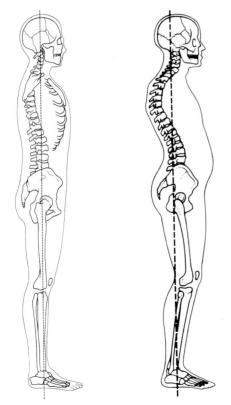

Ideal plumbline alignment
figure A

Kyphosis-Lordosis
figure B

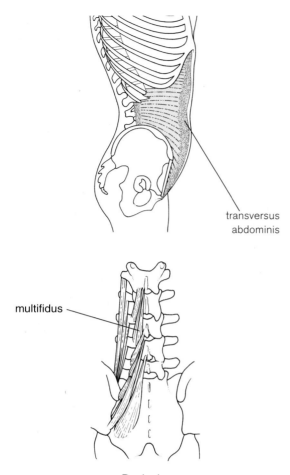

transversus
abdominis

multifidus

Back view
Multifidus. As you 'zip up and hollow' multifidus
is engaged, stabilising your lumbar spine.

Problems arise when these deep stabilising muscles are not working correctly. This can happen when you have the body out of its correct alignment and held in incorrect positions for sustained periods of time ie. if we sit badly for too long. The stabilising muscles are held on a stretch, they weaken, and then other muscles are 'forced' to take over the stabilising role. The wrong muscles are doing the wrong job and there is, therefore, the birth of a faulty recruitment pattern, a pattern of misuse.

In order for a muscle to work efficiently, it needs to be at its optimum length, see Fig 1. When it is held over-stretched or over-lengthened it cannot work effectively, neither will it work properly if it is held over-shortened.

Simply speaking, you can think of muscles as having two types of role: a stabilising role – holding bones in place; or a mobilising role – creating large movements.

In an ideal world muscles designed to stabilise will stabilise, those designed to mobilise will mobilise. Returning to our image of the crane, the stabilisers are the stable base, the mobilisers make the large sweeping movements of the arm of the crane. Some

lumbar spine, ensuring that one vertebra doesn't shear too far off its neighbour – they are the tranversus abdominis, the pelvic floor and a deep back muscle called multifidus.

These muscles engage to form a natural corset, a 'girdle of strength' as Joseph Pilates called it, around your centre so that the movement can take place easily, smoothly and safely. You must have this stable base to support you, in the same way that a tower crane needs a stable base while the long arm moves around.

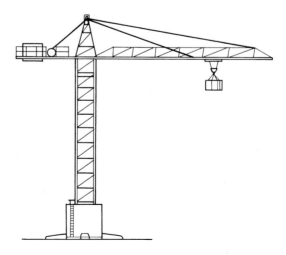

The crane – balancing the body

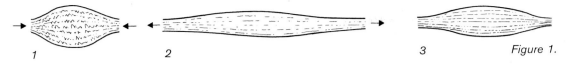

1. *If a muscle is shorter than its ideal length it cannot function effectively*
2. *Longer than its ideal length and it cannot function effectively*
3. *Muscles must be the right length and have the right type of fibres to work effectively*

muscles need to work as stabilisers in some movements and mobilisers in others. If, however, a deep stabilising muscle is not functioning properly due to weakness, a mobiliser may take on a stabilising role, changing its fibre types and meaning that it will no longer be able to work efficiently as a mobiliser.

As an example, your hamstring muscles, which bend and flex the knee, and which for many movements act as mobilising muscles making large movements, are often 'obliged' to take on the stabilising role of stabilising the pelvis because the deep gluteals (buttocks) are too weak. Consequently they tighten and shorten. No amount of stretching will lengthen them while they have to keep stabilising. The solution to this problem would be to strengthen the deep gluteals allowing the hamstrings, at the back of the thighs, to let go!

When these two types of muscles, stabilisers and mobilisers, work perfectly at their own jobs, the body is balanced, all the groups of muscles work in synergy and joints are held in their most favourable position, which is in their natural neutral position. The pitfalls of many fitness programmes are that they target some of the main mobilising muscles with little regard to deep postural muscles. Back to our tower crane, what would happen to that crane if you over-strengthened the arm without equivalent strengthening of the base?

Therein lies the key. You must have good stabilising muscles and sound movement patterns before and while you exercise, especially if you are using gym equipment and weights.

All the exercises in this book are designed to do just this. However, when you see this symbol ↻ next to an exercise, you will know that its main goal is to establish sound movement patterns. Often these exercises look deceptively easy, but don't be fooled. The detailed directions that you are given about the position of your pelvis, shoulders, breathing and engaging the abdominal muscles make it unlike any other fitness technique. It means that you will have to be patient and build your strength gradually. There are no shortcuts! We have to develop your input and output, that is your proprioceptive skills, your kinaesthetic sense, your body awareness, because these lie at the heart of the matter. When you know what you are doing as you move, you will automatically engage the right muscles and the rest will follow.

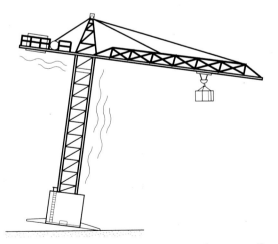

The crane – what would happen to that crane if you over-strengthened the arm without equivalent strengthening of the base?

Joint Mobility 🚴

A joint is simply where two bones meet. There are three main classifications:

• Fibrous joints, which allow for little or no movement, such as the sutures in the skull.

• Cartilaginous joints, which allow for a little movement but offer immense strength, such as the joints between the vertebrae.

• Synovial joints, which are the freely moveable joints, such as the hip and the knee, are the ones we will be targeting.

There are many factors involved in the health of a joint. One of the main factors is its correct alignment. Take a look at the hip joint, for example (Fig A).

The head of the femur or thigh bone is designed to sit snugly in the acetabulum or hip socket. The idea is that the two fit perfectly together, bathed by synovial fluid which keeps the two surfaces well oiled when movement takes place. If, however, let's say through poor posture and muscle imbalance, the joint is held out of alignment, the forces of gravity will no longer fall through the centre of the joint and there will be unnecessary wear and tear on the surfaces,

less lubrication and the potential for arthritis or injury.

Different joints have different movement potential according to their structure. We need therefore to

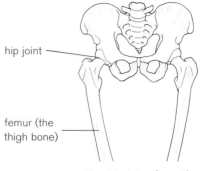

The hip joint (Fig A)

bear in mind which movements are suitable for which joints so that we work within the body's natural movement patterns. If you stress a joint by forcing or twisting it in a direction that is unnatural, you risk weakening or injuring that joint.

Take the hip joint again. We should be able to make the following movements:

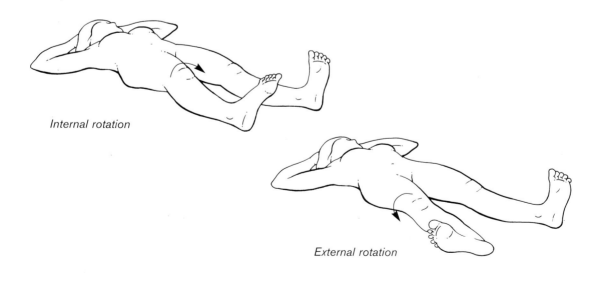

Internal rotation

External rotation

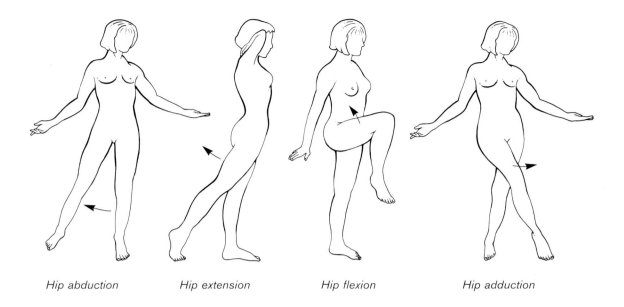

Hip abduction   *Hip extension*   *Hip flexion*   *Hip adduction*

If we lose the ability to make these movements easily we compromise not only the health of the hip joint itself, but our whole body's movement. With the need for hip replacement operations reaching 'epidemic' proportions, clearly we are doing something wrong!

The solution, in a nutshell, is that we need to keep our joints in the best possible natural neutral alignment, supported by strong stabilising muscles and maintaining good muscle balance, enabling the joint to keep its full range of motion so that it can stay well lubricated and healthy. A simple exercise such as Knee Stirs on page 126 will help towards this goal.

By further strengthening the muscles surrounding the hip so that it is well supported, and by keeping the same muscles flexible and the movement patterns sound, you are on the way to maintaining the health of the joint well into your nineties!

Exercises where the main goal is joint mobility will have this symbol 🚲 . Wherever possible, exercises promoting joint mobility should be done before exercises for flexibility as they prepare the body for stretching. Mobility exercises should be performed gently to begin with, as the joint 'opens' you'll find you achieve more movement.

Flexibility

Look up the word flexibility in a dictionary and you will find one definition is 'easily bent', another is 'willing to yield'. Both these should be borne in mind when improving your flexibility by stretching. Technically, flexibility can be defined as the range of movement around a joint or a series of joints such as the spine.

Nothing is more frustrating than working out next to a dancer who effortlessly places her forehead on her knee in a forward bend while you are moving a mere five centimetres forward from the vertical plane – and even that is agony! But you must bear in mind that a variety of factors are going to influence how flexible you are and many of them are out of your control. Above all, stretching should never be competitive. Some of us are just born supple.

Factors that may influence your flexibility:
- The structure and health of the joint.
- The restriction of movement by the surrounding muscles and connective tissue.
- The temperature of the joint and surrounding tissues.
- The elasticity of your muscle tissue.
- The presence of scar tissue.
- The elasticity of your tendons and ligaments.
- The elasticity of your skin.
- Your age.
- Hereditary factors.
- Your gender – females tend to be more flexible.
- The outside temperature.
- The time of day.
- Past injury.
- Fashion – women who regularly wear high heels may find their calf muscles adaptively shorten.
- Your mental approach – can you relax?

Flexibility then is very specific to the individual. It can also be used for different purposes:

Warm-up: Stretching can play a valuable role as part of a warm-up for many activities. These stretches will be 'gentle' in nature and held for a short period of time.

Wind-down: Wind-down stretching at the end of an aerobic or strength training session is a useful way to balance the muscles and reduce the accumulation of lactic acid (a waste product produced in the muscles at the point of fatigue), which can lead to subsequent muscle stiffness.

Developmental stretching: Flexibility may be increased by developmental stretching. We are aiming here for a more permanent change in muscle length, so the stretches can be held for longer and will be more challenging. For this type of stretching it is crucial that the body be thoroughly warmed up, so developmental stretching is ideal after an aerobic session.

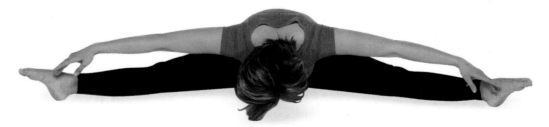

Extreme flexibility

General guidelines for any type of stretching

- Clothes should be comfortable and warm and should not restrict your movements.
- Always ensure that your muscles are warm before they are stretched. Tissues will be more pliable when warm. You will notice that we place the stretches at a point in your workout where you should be nicely warmed up.
- Constantly check your alignment. Joints should normally, but not always, remain in neutral to prevent stress on the joint and to ensure that you isolate the right muscle.
- Be aware of any tension creeping into other parts of the body, especially the neck, jaw, shoulders, calves, feet and hands.
- Use your breathing to help. Initiate the stretch on an out-breath, stabilise and then breathe normally during the stretch, relaxing into it.
- Start the stretch easily and then, if you can, stretch a little further, which will bring you to the developmental part of the stretch.
- A developmental stretch is held for twenty to thirty seconds, released and then repeated two or three times. A warm-up stretch is held for slightly less time.
- Never bounce in a stretch or stretch to the point of pain. This will only bring in a mechanism known as the 'stretch reflex' which is when a nerve responds by signalling the muscle to contract in order to prevent it being injured.
- Although you will be relaxing into the stretch you should always remain in control.
- Recover slowly from a stretch, remembering all your good movement principles.
- A stretch should never be painful. You should feel it, but it should remain a pleasant experience. Any tension should be felt in the muscle itself.
- Be prepared for your body to change from one day to the next.
- Above all enjoy the stretch. If you are not enjoying it, you're not doing it right!

Strength Work

Until very recently, weight training has received a pretty bad press. People have associated it with serious bodybuilding and although it has its own merits, the popular image of 'pumped-up' men and women does not appeal to most of us.

Yet there are many sound reasons for including some weight training in your fitness programme. Joseph Pilates suffered many health problems as a child, including rheumatic fever, rickets and asthma. He saw the benefits of bodybuilding, and used these techniques to rebuild his own strength to the extent that he was eventually used as a model for body-building photographs. The benefits of weight training apply to everyone, whether you are a top international athlete or someone who would just like to adopt a healthier lifestyle.

Recent research has shown that regular weight-bearing exercise can help prevent the onset of osteoporosis and that the earlier we start weight training the better, even in our teens as we are then laying good foundations for the future. About 30 per cent of women and 5 per cent of men suffer from osteoporosis or brittle bone disease. Osteoporosis is defined as a loss of bone mineral leading to thinning of the bone. Although bone looks very solid it is in fact full of holes rather like coral.

Bone health is determined by nutrition, mineral and vitamin content and by the amount of stress it is

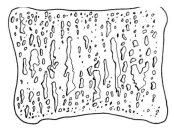

Healthy bone

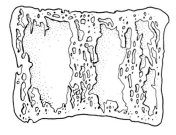

Brittle bone

put under. This is one type of stress that is good for us! Bones are thicker and stronger when they are stressed because stresses produce electrical effects in the bone which, in turn, encourage bone growth. If there is no stress, then the bone will be less dense and weaker. During our lives there is a constant turnover of bone – up until the age of thirty-five we lose as much old bone each year as we make new bone so there is no problem. From that age onwards, however, we tend to lose about 1 per cent of our bone mass each year. When women reach menopause, their bone loss accelerates with an increased loss of 2 per cent per year for up to ten years. By the age of seventy, approximately one third of our bone mass will have been lost.

Bone mass is affected by:

- Hormonal status: menopausal women in particular have an accelerated bone loss which comes with the decline in the ovarian hormone, oestrogen.
- Dietary intake: especially the inclusion of naturally occurring plant oestrogens and calcium in our diet during our growing years.
- Genetic factors: determine the size of our bones and muscles.
- Physical activity: particularly weight-bearing exercise.

So here we have a problem for which we have a readily available prevention! It must be time, therefore, for us all to take note and include some weight-bearing activity in our lives.

It is not just your bones which will benefit from adding weight training to your workout, your muscles will too. From birth until early adulthood, our muscles enlarge as we grow. Unfortunately as we age and our lifestyle becomes less active, we lose muscle mass – in fact some 20–40 per cent by the time we reach the age of eighty. The fibres shrink and are replaced by – guess what? – fat or connective tissue. The central nervous system, which stimulates the fibres, finds it increasingly difficult to get the relevant message through and the muscle is less able to work without fatigue. The beauty of our Pilates Gym™ programme is that we are working not only on the muscles but on the nervous system as well.

We have talked about the medical benefits of using weights, but the aesthetic advantages are to be seen all around us. Impressive body shapes of all proportions are laid before us in the various forms of the media. Despite what anyone will admit, vanity plays its part in all our lives: looking good makes us feel good. Basically it's up to you how much 'tone' you wish to add to your muscles. Adults typically lose approximately 2.5 kilos of lean (muscle) weight, and gain 7 kilos of fat every decade of life. This appears as a 4.5 kilo weight gain on the bathroom scales, but really represents a 9.5 kilo change in body composition. This leads to an increase in percentage of body fat – unattractive and unhealthy.

Taking up cardiovascular exercise can reduce fat weight but will not replace lost muscle tissue. Muscle is very active tissue and our loss of muscle as we age leads to a lower energy requirement and therefore a reduced resting metabolism. In other words we will burn less calories while resting (our resting metabolic rate decreases approximately 2–5 per cent per decade). Regular strength training can improve our body composition through an improvement in muscle tissue and enhance the way we look and feel. The key to a well-balanced programme is to include all three components – strength, cardiovascular exercise and sound nutrition.

We recommend using a range of weights varying from 0.5 to 2.5 kilograms. You may wish to use heavier weights to achieve more definition; this is fine but your technique must be good. Our main concern is that you do not sacrifice flexibility for strength, which is why we include so many stretching exercises to be done alongside the strengthening exercises.

Whenever you see the symbol 🏋️ the primary aim of those exercises will be to strengthen muscles and bones. Remember that strength is the capacity to exert a muscle against resistance. We want to increase this strength progressively, by increasing the:

- Frequency: the time you spend training. Ideally 3–5 times per week.
- Intensity: adding more resistance, that is heavier weights. It is important to understand how inherited physical factors influence your fitness potential. Such knowledge enables you to establish realistic training goals and follow sensible exercise guidelines. Limiting factors include: age, gender, body build, limb strength and muscle length.
- Repetitions: the amount of times you lift a weight. Work between 8-12 repetitions.

General guidelines when using free weights and machine bases

- As our aim is to give a safe and effective foundation to those who are just starting out on the path to a fit and healthy lifestyle, our concern is to establish quality technique first and foremost. Once the seed is sown, there are many places to go as regards the ways in which you can train with weights.
- Ensure that when using a machine, it is set correctly for you.
- Choose a weight that allows you to perform the technique safely and effectively but which, at the same time, provides you with enough resistance to challenge the target muscles. You should be working harder as you progress through your repetitions. For example, during a set of ten repetitions your ninth and tenth should feel as if you are reaching a point of 'failure', where you cannot perform any more quality repetitions because of the increased production of lactic acid. Each individual reaches the point of failure at different times due to varying strengths in certain muscle groups; experience will dictate your personal limits. This is why you should take the time to perfect your technique.
- The number of sets and repetitions you do depends on what you wish to achieve, on what your goals are. For example, lower weights and a high number of repetitions is the general guideline for an endurance athlete e.g. a marathon runner. On the other hand, if you want to increase muscle size lift heavier weights and perform fewer repetitions. Remember that you should always be aiming for a balanced body.
- The following programme should give you that solid base from which to build:

Begin with two sets of eight repetitions for each body part. This will allow you to focus on your technique and alignment. When eight repetitions are performed comfortably (physically and mentally) you can then progress to nine repetitions. When you have worked up to twelve repetitions and your technique and alignment are effective then you can increase the weight. This will keep the emphasis on you working safely and effectively while maintaining all your Pilates Gym™ principles. Build up to three sets on each excercise. To begin with use the three sets in the following ways:

Set One: Establish Sound Movement Patterns. Use a low weight to warm up specific muscle groups. Focus on technique and alignment.

Set Two: Strength. Increase resistance, if possible, maintaining focus and correct technique and alignment.

Set Three: Still with strength in mind. Lower the resistance to ensure maintenance of focus, technique and alignment.

- Always work through the full range of movement.
- Rest between sets for between 30–90 seconds.
- Do not go too fast, too soon. Technique and safety should be uppermost in your mind. Everything else builds from there.
- A word of warning: if you have been used to lifting weights or working out on machines using different techniques to those we are suggesting in this book, you will need to lower the weight or resistance to begin with to give your body time to adapt to the new method. It may be that you have been using different muscle groups or even 'cheating' mechanisms. Give your body time to adjust!

- Ensure that you rest your muscles sufficiently. Muscle soreness may occur after a workout. It is a natural process that is experienced by everyone at some point and is usually experienced on the second day after a session. It is something that occurs at the beginning of a training programme or with the introduction of new exercises. Muscles need rest to recover and develop. Training while a muscle is still sore increases the risk of injury and the effectiveness of the muscle. Adequate rest for each muscle group (usually between forty-eight to seventy-two hours) allows the muscle to recover, gain strength and therefore achieve faster progression and results. Listen to your body. This is a skill that will improve with time and experience. Ideally, use therapies such as massage, sauna, etc to compliment your programme.
- Do not ignore the stretches we will give you to do before, during and after weights sessions. It has been proved that increased flexibility will improve muscle strength and length and decrease the effects of muscle soreness.

Aerobic Work ♡

In the United Kingdom every year over 100,000 people die from heart-related illnesses. Is it not time that we began to look after the heart, the most important muscle in the body?

In order to improve cardiovascular efficiency (the heart and lungs) we must have a programme of aerobic exercise. As our cardiovascular system keeps us alive, justifications for enhancing its efficiency should not be necessary. However, human nature being what it is, we generally consider our health only as a last resort.

The cardiovascular system is our engine and, like the engine of a car, it requires servicing and re-tuning! It dictates our energy levels and performance and along with sound nutrition is essential to our quality of life. The effect on our cardiovascular system can be felt in everyday actions whether we are walking up and down stairs or running for the train.

Combining aerobic exercise with the other elements of our total fitness programme has the following benefits:

- Increases the size of the heart
- Lowers resting heart rate
- Increases blood supply to the heart and rest of the body
- Lowers the risk of heart disease
- Lowers blood pressure
- Improves lung function
- Lowers body-fat content
- Improves muscle tone
- Increases the resistance to fatigue
- Improves general appearance
- Improves self-image and self-esteem
- Improves ability to relax
- Improves mental alertness

The increasing coverage in the media, the explosion of health clubs and an increase in public awareness has shown that, although aerobics classes rightly have their place, there are now many alternatives to suit the individual. Once your aerobic fitness has increased you may want to progress to activities such as outdoor running or cycling, swimming, spinning classes or even a kick-boxing class. Basically, keep yourself interested and motivated by continually developing both your strength and aerobic training.

Examples of aerobic exercise:

Brisk/power walking

Jogging (treadmill/outdoor)

Swimming

Cycling (stationary/outdoor)

Rollerblading

Spinning (instructor-led class)

Kick-boxing

Aerobics class

Cross trainer (machine)

Rowing (indoor/outdoor)

General guidelines for aerobic exercise

- Have a check-up with a doctor before embarking on any exercise programme.
- Choose an activity or class to suit your level of fitness, physical limitations and needs. Find out as much information as you can beforehand, by reading and by talking to qualified and experienced people.
- Use a heart-rate monitor where possible (they are very easy to use). Exercising at the correct intensity is essential to ensure safe and effective training.
- Do not go too fast too soon. Build your fitness steadily and progressively. Work at your own level. If you have a low level of aerobic fitness start with moderate exercise such as walking, stationary cycling or swimming.
- Ideally we should exercise aerobically for a minimum of twenty minutes, three to five times per week. However, we all have varying fitness levels so set yourself a manageable programme to start with. If you set yourself too high a goal and your fitness levels are low then the chances are you will fail and give your motivation an unnecessary blow. Be sensibly progressive. As your fitness improves, increase the duration and intensity of your training while still monitoring your heart rate.
- Avoid carrying unnecessary tension, especially in your shoulders. Relax and monitor your breathing.
- Allow your body to rest. Have at least two days off from exercise per week. There is a fine line between training and over-training.
- Ensure that you are using the correct footwear especially when running. Incorrect footwear can lead to conditions such as shin splints and ankle injuries.

How To Use This Book

The aim of this book, therefore, is to introduce you to an alternative way of exercising. In order to understand this new approach, you will need to learn the methods discussed in the chapter headed 'The Golden Rules'. It is vital that you do not proceed until you have mastered these techniques.

Once you are familiar with the skills taught in 'The Golden Rules', you can start the exercise programmes. We have given you two programmes. One for when you workout at the gym, the other for when you are at home. Learn the exercises, then you can start varying your workouts, combining different types of exercise to keep the balance of the body but also to avoid the trap of going over the same routine each day.

And, above all, have fun.

Before You Begin

It is always wise to consult your doctor before you take up a new exercise regime. Whenever you workout please do not exercise if you:

- Are feeling unwell.
- Have just eaten a heavy meal.
- Have been drinking alcohol.
- Are in pain from an injury – always consult your practitioner first, as rest may be needed before you exercise.
- Have taken painkillers, as it will mask any warning pains.
- Are undergoing medical treatment, or are taking drugs – again, you will need to consult your medical practitioner first.

Please note: not all of the exercises are suitable for use during pregnancy. If you have a back problem you will need to consult your medical practitioner.

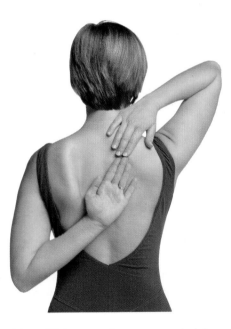

Many Pilates exercises are wonderful for back-related problems, but you should always get expert guidance

Working Out in a Gym

There has never been such a wide choice of fitness clubs and leisure centres as there is today. Many things will influence you in your choice, including location, cost, classes and whether friends are existing members. Here are a few guidelines to help you make your choice:

- Look out for staff qualifications. They should be on display in the reception or gym area. If not, do not be afraid to ask to see certificates. If in doubt you can always check these with one of the fitness industry's professional bodies (see contact details at the back of the book).
- Talk to the fitness staff and do not be afraid to ask questions, for example, 'Do I have a fitness assessment on joining the gym?' – a reputable gym will always provide one.
- There should be a good range of cardiovascular and strength equipment.
- Wear comfortable clothing that does not restrict your movements but that is practical, bearing in mind that you will be using equipment and therefore it should not be too loose and flowing. Also bear in mind that you will be doing some aerobic work, which may be followed by slower exercises, so layers that you can put on and take off are a good idea.
- Wear good-quality training shoes in good condition. Some exercises require you to keep your shoes on, for others you will need to take them off. We have tried to group the exercises so that you are not constantly putting them on and off!

Working Out at Home

- Be sure that you have no pressing, unfinished business.
- Take the telephone off the hook, or put the answering machine on.
- You may prefer silence, otherwise put on some unobtrusive classical, new-age or 'chill out' music.
- All exercises should be done on a padded mat.
- Wear something warm and comfortable, allowing free movement.
- Barefoot is best, non-slip socks otherwise.
- The best time to exercise is in the late afternoon or evening when your muscles are already warmed up as a result of the day's activity. Exercising in the morning is fine, but you will need to take longer to warm-up thoroughly.
- You will need space to work in – you cannot keep stopping to move furniture.
- Items you may need include a mat, a chair, a small flat but firm pillow for under your head or perhaps a folded towel, a larger pillow, a long scarf and a tennis ball.
- You may wish to use hand-held weights and leg weights, and we have given you advice on how to make your own, see page 141.

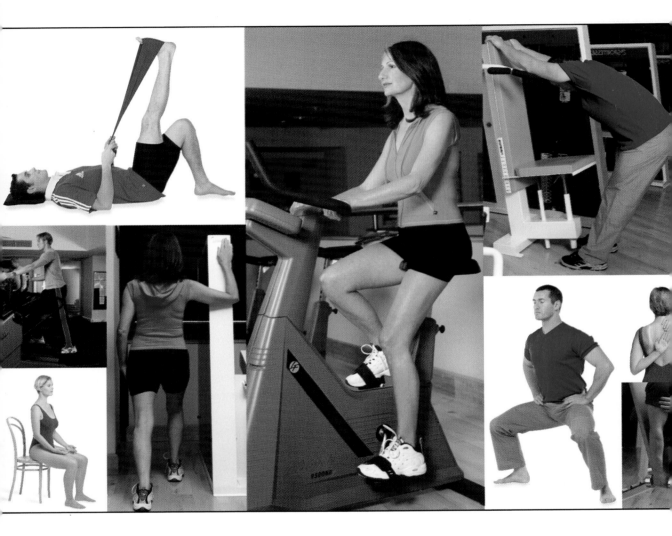

The Six Golden Rules

1. Be prepared
2. Stay focused
3. Stay aligned
4. Breathe right
5. Use your Girdle of Strength
6. Keep the balance

Be Prepared

Whether you are a top athlete about to run the 100 metres at the Olympics or whether you just enjoy a regular workout at the local gym, you will need to prepare yourself for the event or session ahead. Skip your warm-up preparation and you not only risk injury, but you will not get the full benefit of the workout.

There are two elements involved in a good warm-up session:

Mental preparation: you are entering a different zone now. The outside world needs to be left where it is – outside. Bring your focus from outside to inside yourself. Notice any unwanted tension in your body – concentrate on releasing that tension (see page 27 for some good relaxing techniques). You are aiming to be relaxed but ready for action.

Body preparation: we have given you several exercises as part of your warm-up routine. Their aim is to remind you of good movement technique, to re-establish sound movement patterns, to mobilise stiff joints and to ease out any tight muscles gently. We will be giving you stronger, more developmental stretches later in the Pilates Gym™ programme when your body is warmer.

Stay Focused

Now that your focus is within, it needs to stay there! There is no point in concentrating for the first five minutes and then being distracted the first time an attractive body floats by! Do not let your attention wander to the thumping music or the TV screens, it must stay on what you are doing. If you wish to check out the scenery, arrive five minutes before or stay five minutes longer but, for the whole time that you are exercising, only one person matters and that's you and how you are moving. Stay in the zone!

Remember: 'It is the mind itself which builds the body'. As we progress into our new millennium, more and more research is being done into the effect the mind has over the body, so use its power to achieve your goals.

All exercise should involve both mental and physical conditioning: it should train both the mind and the body. Awareness of what you are doing and how you are doing it at all times is central to this

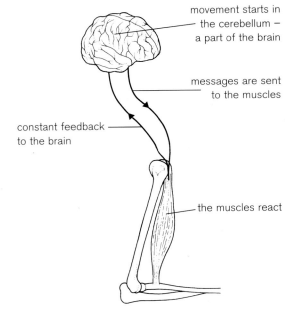

movement starts in the cerebellum – a part of the brain

messages are sent to the muscles

constant feedback to the brain

the muscles react

The two-way communication channel between brain and muscles is just like a telephone line

method. We have already seen the importance of the constant input and output, the two-way communication channel between the brain and muscles.

Just like a telephone line, if there is no activity on the line for a long period, the chances are you'll get cut off! Pilates requires you to be constantly aware of how you are moving, it requires you to focus your mind on each and every movement that you make.

It develops your body's sensory feedback or kinaesthetic sense, so that you know where you are in space and what you are doing with every part of your body. Although some movements themselves may become automatic with time, you still have to concentrate because there is always a further level of awareness to reach, adding layer on layer.

Stay Aligned

So, you are now both mentally and physically prepared to workout. Our next step is to bring the body into good postural alignment. By constantly reminding the body of how it should be standing, sitting or lying and by moving correctly you can gradually start to bring it back into better alignment. This, as we have seen, is essential if we are going to restore the muscle balance in the body. If you exercise without due attention to the correct position of the joints, you risk stressing the joint and building imbalance into the surrounding muscles. You must have your bones in the right place to get the right muscles working. In that way you build the muscles so that they will support the joint and not stress it.

The following exercises are designed to help you correct your postural alignment.

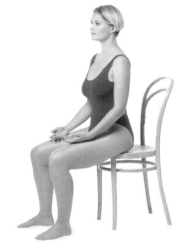

By reminding the body of how it should be standing, sitting or lying you can start to bring it back into better alignment

The Compass
(Finding Pelvic and Spinal Neutral) ↻

Aim

To find the neutral position of the pelvis and the spine.

Starting Position

- Lie on your back with your knees bent, feet hip-width apart and in parallel. You may like a flat firm pillow under your head to allow your neck to maintain its natural curves and stay lengthened and released. This is the Relaxation Position.

- Imagine that you have a compass on your lower abdomen, the navel is north, the pubic bone south, with west and east on either side.

We are going to look at two incorrect positions in order to find the correct one.

Action

1. Tilt your pelvis up towards north – while doing so, the pelvis will 'tuck under'. Notice what has happened to your waist, your hips and your tailbone (coccyx). The waist is flattened, you've

pushed it into the floor, the curve is lost. You have gripped the muscles around your hips and your tailbone has lifted off the floor.

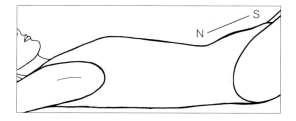

2. Now, carefully (avoid this bit if you have a back injury), move the pelvis so that it is tilting towards south. Notice again what has happened. The low back is arched and feels vulnerable,

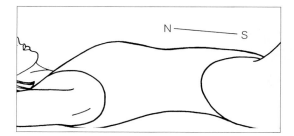

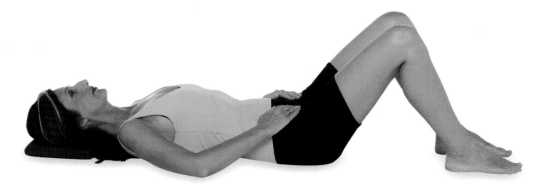

The Relaxation Position

your ribs have flared, you probably have two chins and your stomach is sticking out.

3. Come back to the Starting Position.

We are aiming for a neutral position between the two extremes, neither to north nor south, neither tucked nor arched. Back with the image of the compass, the pointer is level like a spirit level. The tailbone remains down on the floor and lengthens away. Your pubic bone and the prominent bones of your pelvis (arterial/superior iliac spines) are now level.

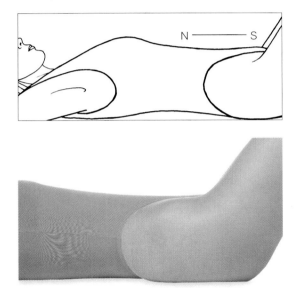

There remains a small natural arch in your back. This is neutral, and all the exercises should be performed in this neutral position unless you are told otherwise. You should learn to recognise your natural neutral position in standing, lying, sitting and side-lying. You would not start your car if the gears were not in neutral, so please do not start an exercise out of neutral!

Be particularly vigilant when you are engaging the lower abdominals (see below) as there is a temptation to tilt or tuck the pelvis. If you are lying down, you can always try placing your hand under your waist – you will then feel if you are pushing the spine into the floor. You want to avoid this.

It is also worth pointing out that if you have a large bottom, you will have more of a hollow in the lumbar region – this does not necessarily mean that you have arched your back. Learn to recognise your natural curve.

Bear in mind too that we also want the pelvis to be level 'west to east'. Many people suffer from a twisted pelvis: the pelvis can be rotated forward on one side as well as tilted. You need to be constantly aware that the pelvis stays neutral, level and stable while you exercise if the right muscles are to work. Of course, once we add movements into the programme the pelvis will sometimes move out of neutral, e.g. with Roll Downs.

Please note, though, that occasionally, if the muscles around the pelvis are very out of balance, you may find neutral very difficult to maintain. When this is the case, we usually recommend that you consult your practitioner as it is often necessary to work in the best neutral you can achieve. Usually after a few months, as the muscles begin to rebalance, neutral becomes more comfortable.

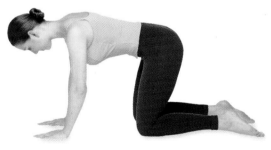

On all fours

Alignment in Standing ↻

The following checklist should help you align your body correctly while standing:

Keep your shoulder blades down into your back.

Check your pelvis — is it in neutral?

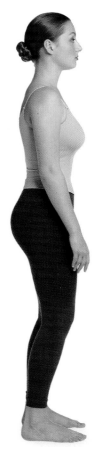

Imagine a balloon attached to the top of your head pulling you up.

Allow your neck to release.

Keep your breastbone soft.

Keep your elbows open.

Lengthen up through the spine.

When you bend your knees, they should bend directly over the centre of your foot.

Keep the weight even on both feet — do not allow them to roll in or out.

Head, Neck and Shoulder Alignment ↻

One last word about the alignment of your head, neck and shoulders. Throughout the book you will notice that we give you instructions to keep the shoulder blades down, the upper body open and the neck released. We will also be directing you, especially when you are using the machine bases, to keep your chin tucked in gently. This action engages the deep neck flexors that stabilise the cervical spine. The action is subtle and, to get it right, you should practise it in the Relaxation Position.

Neck Rolls/Chin Tucks ↻

Aim

To release tension in the neck. To learn how to stabilise the neck.

Starting Position

- Lie in the Relaxation Position, with your knees bent and your arms resting on your lower abdomen. Use a flat pillow for this if you are uncomfortable without .

Action

1. Release your neck. Release your jaw, allow your tongue to widen at its base.
2. Keep the neck nicely lengthened. Soften your breastbone and allow the shoulder blades to widen and melt into the floor.
3. Now, allow your head to roll *slowly* to one side.
4. Bring it back to the centre and over to the other side. Just let your head roll slowly from side to side. Do not rush, take your time.

5. When the neck feels free, bring the head to the centre and gently tuck your chin in, keeping the head on the floor and lengthening out of the back of the neck. Imagine that you are holding a ripe peach under your chin – you need to hold it fast, but mustn't crush its delicate skin!
6. Return the head to the centre.
7. Repeat the rolling to the side and chin tuck eight times.

Watchpoints

- Do not force the head or neck, just let them roll naturally.
- Do not lift your head off the floor when you tuck the chin in.
- If you find your jaw becomes tense as you tuck your chin in, gently place the tip of your tongue on the roof of your mouth behind your front teeth as you lengthen through the back of the neck.

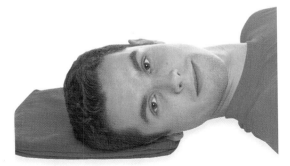 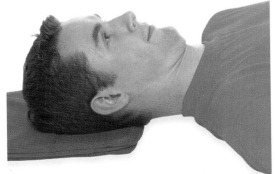

Breathe Right

Hopefully, you are now mentally and physically prepared and aligned, so we wish to concentrate next on improving the efficiency of your breathing.

The most efficient breathing technique is called 'lateral thoracic breathing', which involves breathing wide and full into your back and sides. This makes sound sense as our lungs are situated in the ribcage, so, by expanding the ribcage, the volume of the cavity and the resultant capacity for oxygen intake are increased. It also encourages us to make maximum use of the lower part of our lungs. This type of breathing also works the muscles between the ribs, facilitating their expansion and making the upper body more fluid and mobile. Your lungs become like bellows, the lower ribcage expanding wide as you breathe in and closing down as you breathe out. The diaphragm moves down as you breathe in. We do not wish to block its descent but, rather, encourage the movement to be widthways and into the back.

To practise, try the following:

1. Sit or stand. Wrap a scarf, towel or stretch band around your ribs, crossing it over at the front.

2. Holding the opposite ends of the scarf and gently pulling it tight, breathe in and allow your ribs to expand the scarf. As you breathe out, you may gently squeeze the scarf to help you empty your lungs fully and relax the ribcage. Allow the breastbone to soften. Try to keep your upper shoulders calm as you do this.

This type of breathing is important to our way of exercising, as is also the timing of the breath because you can help or hinder a movement by breathing in or out. As a general rule, the most effective way to breathe while exercising is to:

* Breathe in to prepare for a movement.

* Breathe out to stabilise (see below) as you move or make an action.

* Breathe in, still stabilised, to recover.

Moving on the exhalation will enable you to relax into the movement and prevent you from tensing. It also offers you greater core stability at the hardest part of the exercise and safeguards against you holding your breath, which can unduly stress the heart and lead to serious complications.

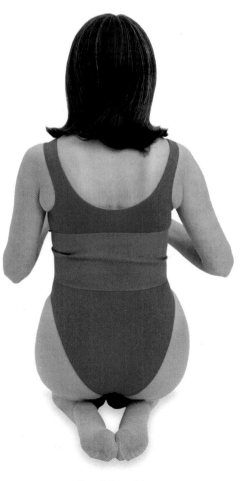

Scarf breathing

Use Your Girdle of Strength (Core Stability)

This, the creation of a girdle of strength, is at the centre of Pilates and involves learning how to stabilise the lumbar spine, the pelvis and the shoulder blades on the ribcage. You must master these skills before moving on.

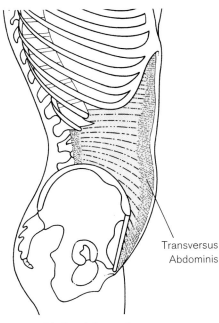

Girdle of Strength

Transversus Abdominis

It is fascinating to think that over eighty years ago Joseph Pilates discovered that if he hollowed his navel back towards his spine, his low back felt protected. He had no medical knowledge of this 'core stability' or the tranversus abdominis muscle, but he had superb body awareness and thus introduced the direction 'navel to spine' into all Pilates exercises.

We have moved on since then. The latest medical research indicates that the best stability is to be had if the action begins with engaging the pelvic floor muscles and then engaging the lower abdominals. This is why we now use the direction 'zip up and hollow': as you breathe out you draw up the muscles of the pelvic floor as if you are doing up this internal zip and then hollow the lower abdominals back to the spine!

You will notice that we have chosen to use the word 'hollow' to describe the action. It is very important that you do not grip your abdominals tightly as this will only create unnecessary tension and you will probably engage the wrong muscles to boot. Remember that because stabilising muscles are postural muscles, they need to be worked at approximately 25 per cent of their full capability (Maximum Voluntary Contraction) so that you build endurance into the muscles.

Each of the following exercises should be practised regularly to ensure that you are stabilising correctly and not 'cheating' in any way!

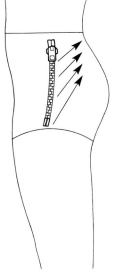

'Zip up and hollow' drawing up and in the muscles of the pelvic floor and hollowing the lower abdomen back towards the spine

The Pelvic Elevator ↻

Aim

To isolate and engage the deep stabilising muscles of the pelvis and spine – tranversus abdominis, pelvic floor and multifidus.

In order to achieve the best possible stability, you need to be able to contract the pelvic floor at the same time as hollowing the lower abdominals to engage tranversus abdominis.

It is not easy to isolate and engage the pelvic floor and it takes considerable concentration. We are talking about the urethra in men and women and the muscles of the vagina for women. At this stage, we do not want you to engage the muscles around the anus, the back passage, as it is too easy for the buttock muscles to kick in and substitute.

We know it sounds daft but one way to help locate these muscles is to suck your thumb as you draw them up inside. Crazy, but effective! Guys, you should think of lifting your 'crown jewels' or your 'tackle'!

Once you have found the pelvic floor muscles, it should be easier to isolate the tranversus abdominis. To engage tranversus correctly, that is at no more than 25 per cent, think of:
- Hollowing
- Scooping
- Drawing back the abdominals towards the spine
- Sucking in

The Elevator in Sitting ↻

Starting Position
- Sit on an upright chair.
- Make sure that you are sitting square with the weight even on both buttocks.
- Imagine that your pelvic floor is like the lift in a building. This exercise requires you to take the 'lift' up to different floors of the building.

Action
1. Breathe in wide and full to your back and your sides and lengthen up through the spine.
2. As you breathe out, draw up the muscles of your pelvic floor as if you are trying to stop the flow of urine and take the pelvic 'lift' up to the first floor of the building.
3. Breathe in and release the 'lift' back to the ground floor.

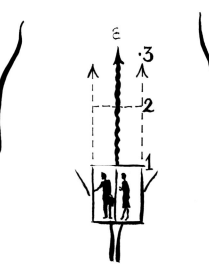

The Pelvic Elevator

4. Breathe out and now take the lift up to the second floor of the building; most people feel their lower abdominals engage.
5. Breathe in and release.
6. Breathe out and take the lift up to the third floor. Breathe in and relax.

Watchpoints

Everyone is different, but for most people when you reach the first to second floor, you feel the deep lower abdominals engage. This is tranversus coming into play. By starting the action from underneath, you encourage the 'six-pack' muscle to stay quiet. If you were to take the lift all the way to the top floor, you would probably be engaging the muscles at over 40 per cent and the rectus abdominis would take over – so keep the action low and gentle.

- Do not allow the buttock muscles to join in.
- Keep your jaw relaxed.
- Don't take your shoulders up to the top floor too – keep them down and relaxed.
- Try not to grip around your hips.
- Keep the pelvis and spine quite still.

Once you have found your pelvic floor muscles you need to learn how to engage them in lots of different positions. The instructions we will give you from now on will be 'zip up and hollow'. You need to imagine that you have an internal zip from your pelvic floor up and hollow lower abdominals back to the spine.

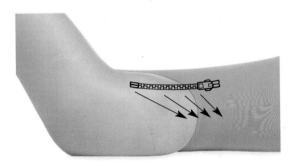

Zip up and hollow

The following three positions will help to ensure that no cheating goes on.

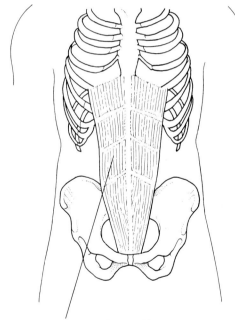

The rectus abdominis (six-pack)

Most fitness techniques focus on strengthening rectus abdominis (the six-pack). This is a superficial muscle which does not have a primary stabilising role and it can often become over-dominant.

Stabilising on All Fours ↺

Action

1. Kneel on all fours, your hands beneath your shoulders and shoulder-width apart.
2. Your knees are beneath your hips. Have the top of your head lengthening away from your tail-bone. Your pelvis and spine are in neutral.
3. Breathe in to prepare.
4. Breathe out, and zip up and hollow the lower abdominals up towards the spine. Your back should not move.
5. Breathe in and release.

You may like to try this in your underwear over a mirror to check that you are keeping the actions low and gentle. It should be easy to spot if your six-pack muscle is dominating the action – which of course we wish to avoid.

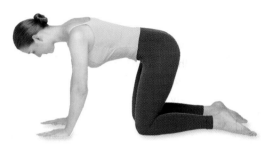

On all fours

Stabilising in Prone-lying ↺

Action

1. Lie on your front. Rest your head on your folded hands, opening the shoulders out and relaxing the upper back – you may need a small, flat cushion under your abdomen if your low back is uncomfortable. Your legs are shoulder-width apart and relaxed.
2. Breathe in to prepare, breathe out and zip up and hollow and lift the lower abdominals off the floor. Imagine there is a precious egg under them that must not be crushed. Do not tighten the buttocks.
3. Breathe in and release. Again there should be no movement in the pelvis or spine.

This, then, is your strong centre and, for most of the exercises, you will be asked to zip up and hollow before and while you move, your movements lengthening away from a strong centre.

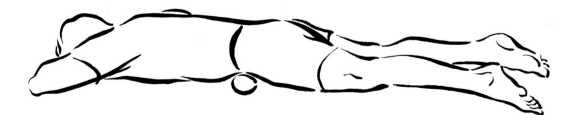

Precious egg

Stabilising in the Relaxation Position ↻

Action

1. Lie on your back with your knees bent, hip-width apart and in parallel. Check that your pelvis is in neutral. Place your hands on your pelvis, find your prominent pelvic bones (anterior and superior iliac spines). Put your fingertips on these bones, then move them two centimetres inwards and five centimetres downwards. Very, very gently feel your deep abdominals. Do not do this if you have abdominal problems or if it causes you discomfort.

2. Breathe in to prepare.

3. Breathe out, zip up and hollow the lower abdominals back towards the spine. You should feel the deep muscles under your fingers engage and become firm, a bit like the seatbelt in a plane being wrapped round you. If the muscles are recruited correctly they will stay scooped out and not bulge out at all. *Do not allow the pelvis to tuck under.* Do not push into the spine. Keep your tailbone on the floor and lengthening away.

4. Breathe in and relax.

When you can do this easily, practise zipping up and hollowing for both the in- and the out-breath. Use lateral thoracic breathing, wide and full into your sides and back and stay zipped.

You must be careful not to tuck the pelvis under, that is tilting it to north. If you do, you will lose your neutral position (see above) and it means that other muscles – the rectus abdominis and the hip flexors – are cheating and doing the work instead of the transversus and internal obliques. If you are comfortable with your hand under your waist you can check to see that you are not pushing into the spine.

Once you have learned to create a strong centre, you can then add movements such as rotation, flexion and extension. The exercises given on page 34–6 will take you through this step by step.

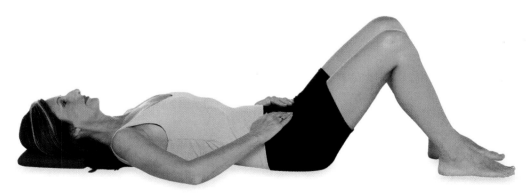

The Relaxation Position

Pelvic Stability –
Leg Slides, Drops, Folds and Turnout ↻

Aim

To learn how to keep the pelvis neutral and stable while the limbs are moved.

Now that you have mastered the breathing, correct alignment, the creation of a strong centre and how to isolate the stabilising muscles, we need to learn to add movement and the ability to co-ordinate all this. It isn't easy to begin with but, as with learning to ride a bicycle, it will soon become automatic. Meanwhile, the process of learning this co-ordination is fabulous mental and physical training as it stimulates that two-way communication between the brain and the muscles – real mind-body exercises. We usually start with small movements, and then build up to more complicated combinations. Here, we have given you four movements to practise, all of them requiring you to keep the pelvis completely still. A useful image to use is that you have a set of car headlights on your pelvis shining up at the ceiling. The beam should be fixed and not mimicking searchlights! You can vary which exercises you practise at each session. The Starting Position is the same for all three.

Starting Position for Pelvic Stability Exercises

- Adopt the Relaxation Position.
- Check that your pelvis is in neutral, tailbone down and lengthening away.
- Place your hands on your pelvic bones to check for unwanted movement.

Action for LEG SLIDES

1. Breathe in wide and full to prepare.
2. Breathe out, zip up and hollow and slide one leg away along the floor, keeping the lower abdominals engaged and the pelvis still, stable, and in neutral.
3. Breathe into your lower ribcage while you return the leg to the bent position, trying to keep the stomach hollow. If you cannot yet breathe in and maintain a strong centre, then take an extra breath and return the leg on the out-breath.
4. Repeat five times with each leg.

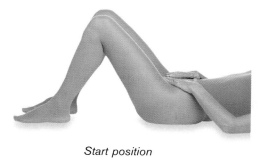

Start position

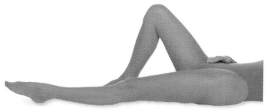

Leg slid away

Action for KNEE DROPS

1. Breathe in wide and full to prepare.
2. Breathe out, zip up and hollow and slowly allow one knee to open to the side. Go only so far as the pelvis stays still.

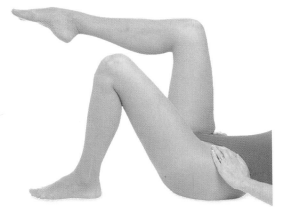

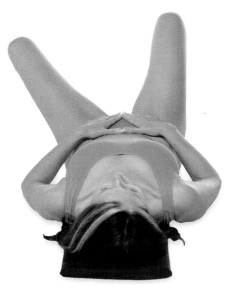

Knee Drop

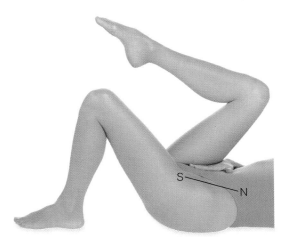

Knee Fold

down into the hip and anchoring there. Do not lose your neutral pelvis, the tailbone stays down. Do not rely on the other leg to stabilise you. Imagine your foot is on a large chocolate eclair, you don't want to press down on it.

3. Breathe in and hold.
4. Breathe out, zipped up and hollowed, as you return the foot slowly to the floor.
5. Repeat five times with each leg.

3. Breathe in, still zipped up and hollowed, as the knee returns to the centre.
4. Repeat five times with each leg.

Action for KNEE FOLDS

With this movement it is particularly useful to feel that the muscles stay 'scooped' and do not bulge while you fold the knee in, so you may like to find your pelvic bones again and move your fingers two centimetres inwards and five centimetres down-wards. Very gently, feel the muscles engage as you zip up and hollow.

1. Breathe in wide and full to prepare.
2. Breathe out, zip up and hollow and fold the right knee up, think of the thigh bone dropping

Incorrect Knee Fold. The pelvis has tilted north

Action for TURNING OUT THE LEG

This next action involves turning the leg out from the hip; as you do so you are working your deep gluteal muscles, especially gluteus medius which is one of the main stabilising muscles of the pelvis.

Please take advice if you suffer from sciatica.

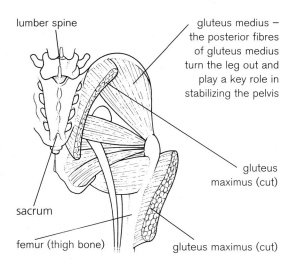

lumber spine

gluteus medius – the posterior fibres of gluteus medius turn the leg out and play a key role in stabilizing the pelvis

gluteus maximus (cut)

sacrum

femur (thigh bone)

gluteus maximus (cut)

The pelvis (back view)

Follow steps 1. and 2. for Knee Folds.

3. Breathe out, zip up and hollow and turn the right leg out from the hip bringing, if you can, the foot to touch the left knee. Do not allow the pelvis to tilt or twist or turn, keep it central and stable. Headlights glued to the ceiling please!

4. Breathe in, and then out, zip up and hollow, as you reverse the movement to return the foot to the floor.

5. Repeat five times to each side.

Watchpoints

- Remember that you are trying to avoid even the slightest movement of the pelvis.
- It helps to think of the waist being long and even on both sides as you make the movement.

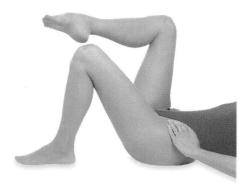

Turning out the leg

- Try to keep your neck and jaw released throughout. If you feel tension creeping in, do a few Standing Adductor Stretches page 61 and Neck Rolls page 27.

Try

Another way to test that your pelvis is remaining still and stable is to place both your hands evenly under your waist. This should feel comfortable and should not alter your neutral position.

As you stabilise and slide, drop or fold the leg you should be able to feel any unwanted movement with your hands.

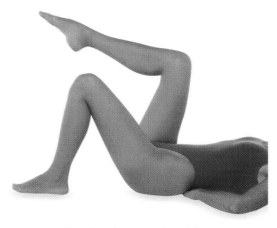

Keeping the neutral position

Scapular Stability

The final part of our Girdle of Strength involves learning how to stabilise the shoulder blades. We have been concentrating up until now on the lower half of the body. We also need to learn how to move the upper body correctly, with good mechanics. For this, we need to find the muscles (lower trapezius and serratus anterior) which set the shoulder blades down into the back, holding them in just the right position to allow the arm to move freely and easily with the shoulder joint correctly positioned.

To find these muscles, try the following exercise.

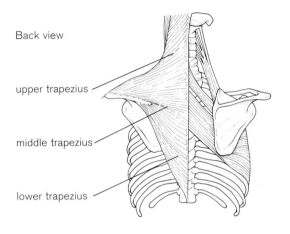

Back view

upper trapezius

middle trapezius

lower trapezius

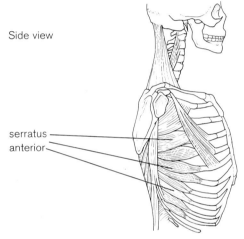

Side view

serratus anterior

The Dart Stage One ↻

Aim

To locate the muscles that stabilise the shoulder blades.

Starting Position

* Lie on your front. You may place a flat pillow under your forehead to allow you to breathe.
* Your arms are down by your sides, your palms facing your body. Your neck is long. Your legs are relaxed but in parallel.

Action

1. Breathe in to prepare, lengthen through the spine and gently tuck your chin in.
2. Breathe out, zip up and hollow and pull your shoulder blades down into your back, lengthening your fingers away from you down towards your feet. The top of your head stays lengthening away.
3. Keep looking straight down at the floor. Do not tip your head back.
4. Breathe in and feel the length of the body from the tips of your toes to the top of your head.
5. Breathe out, still zipping up, and release.

Watchpoints

* Keep hollowing the lower abdominals.
* Do not strain the neck. It should feel released as your shoulders engage down into your back. Think of a swan's neck growing out between its wings.
* Please remember to keep your feet on the floor.
* Please stop if you feel at all uncomfortable in the low back.

Moving On

The muscles which you felt pulling your shoulder blades down into your back are the stabilising muscles. Now that you have located them, try to feel them working in this next exercise.

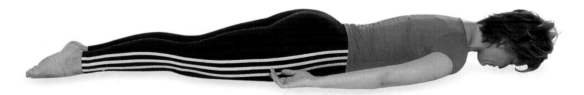

Start position

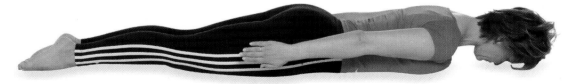

Full position

Floating Arms ↻

Aim

To learn correct upper-body mechanics.

Starting Position

- Stand correctly – see page 26.
- Now place your right hand on your left shoulder, the idea being that your hand checks that the upper part of your trapezius muscle remains 'quiet' for as long as possible. Very often this part will overwork, so think of it staying soft and released, while the lower trapezius below your shoulder blades works to set the shoulder blades down into your back.

Action

1. Breathe in to prepare and lengthen up through the spine, letting the neck be free.
2. Breathe out, zipping up and hollowing and slowly begin to raise the left arm, reaching wide out of the shoulder blades like a bird's wing. Think of the hand as leading the arm, the arm following the hand as it floats upwards. You will need to rotate the arm so that the palm opens to the ceiling as the arm reaches shoulder level. Try to keep the shoulder under your right hand still with the shoulder blades dropping down into your back as long as possible.
3. Breathe in as you lower the arms to your sides.
4. Repeat three times with each arm.

Watchpoints

- Keep a sense of openness in the upper body.
- Do not allow your upper body to shift to the side, keep centred.

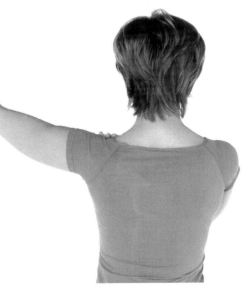

Start position

Full position

The Starfish ↻

We need now to combine everything we have learned.

The Starfish Stage One: The Upper Body

Starting Position
- Lie in the Relaxation Position, this time having your arms down by your sides.

Action
1. Breathe in wide into your lower ribcage to prepare.
2. Breathe out, zip up and hollow and start to take one arm above you in a backstroke movement as if to touch the floor – you may not be able to touch the floor easily so only move the arm as far as is comfortable. Do not force the arm, keep it soft and open with the elbow bent. The shoulder blade stays down into your back. The ribs stay calm. Do not allow the back to arch at all.
3. Breathe in as you return the arms to your sides.
4. Repeat five times with each arm.

Please note: not everyone can touch the floor behind without arching the upper back. Do not strain – it is better to keep the back down than force the arm.

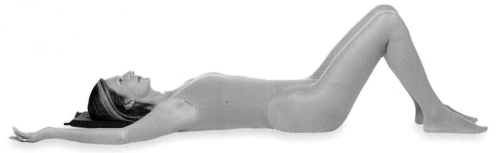

Arm above head – keep the shoulder blades down

The Full Starfish

Now we are going to co-ordinate the opposite arm and leg movement away from the strong centre. Although this looks simple, it is a sophisticated movement pattern, using all the skills of good movement we have learned so far. It is the base on which we will build the whole fitness programme.

Starting Position
- As for The Starfish Stage One.

Action
1. Breathe in wide and full to prepare.
2. Breathe out, zip up and hollow and slide the

right leg away along the floor and take the left arm above you in a backstroke movement. Keep the pelvis completely neutral, stable and still and the stomach muscles engaged. Keep a sense of width and openness in the upper body and shoulders, and try to keep the shoulder blades down into your back and the ribcage calm.

3. Breathe in, still zipped up and hollowed, and return the limbs to the Starting Position.

4. Repeat five times, alternating arms and legs.

Watchpoints
- Do not be tempted to over-reach. The girdle of strength must stay in place.
- Slide the leg in a line with the hip.

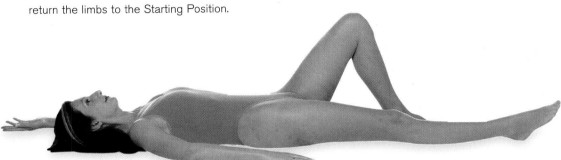

Full stretch

Keep the Balance

We have added balance as the last of our Golden Rules as we want you to be aware throughout your workout of the balance within your body. A body must be balanced in order to move normally. The word balance here refers to maintaining the right muscle balance around a joint. For example, too many repetitions of the Leg Press could over-develop your quadriceps (front of your thighs) at the expense of your hamstrings. Do not become obsessed with one muscle or muscle group. The Pilates Gym™ programme should help to avoid this pitfall.

You must also balance strength and flexibility. Your body sacrifices one for the other so if you overdevelop a muscle you risk it becoming less flexible. To move normally, you need a body which is both supple and strong. With this in mind, we have given you stretches to do between strengthening weight or resistance work.

And last but not least, pay attention to including all the 'ingredients' in the programme. This doesn't mean that you have to go to the gym or use weights at home, but you should be aware that your body needs some type of strength training to maintain the health of your bones and the tone of your muscles. Adapt the programme to suit your needs but do not ignore any of the essential ingredients or 'the cake' won't turn out right!

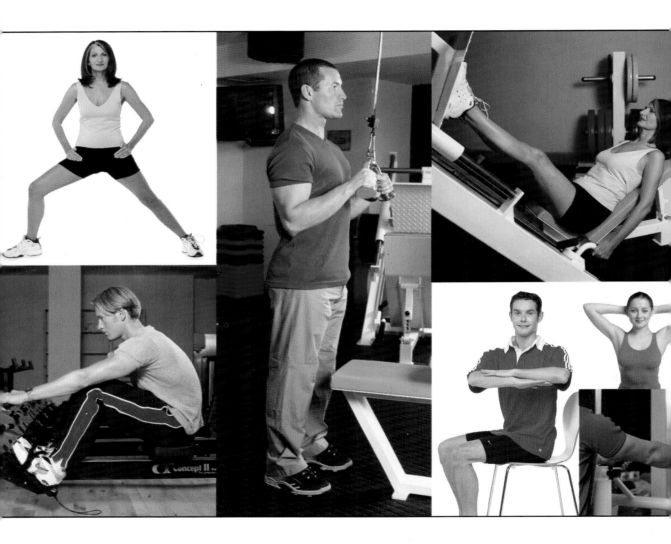

Working Out at the Gym

In this section we are going to show you how to apply the Six Golden Rules to your gym workout. They are:

- Be prepared
- Stay focused
- Stay aligned
- Breathe right
- Use your Girdle of Strength
- Keep the balance

If you are a regular gym goer you will probably already have a routine which you follow. We will be suggesting new combinations, new exercise, a whole new approach to the way you normally workout.

Not only will you now be paying attention to alignment, breathing and stability, but you may have to change the order you usually use the machine bases, add extra stretches, as well as including Pilates exercises to balance the body. It is very important that you do not attempt the same weight or resistance that you used to work at because your technique will have changed. Lighten the load until you are familiar with the new approach.

If you have never set foot inside a gym before you will need to get expert advice from the gym staff on how their machines work. Then you can apply our principles.

On page 111, Gym Workouts, you will find advice as to how best to combine aerobic work, the machine bases, abdominal work, etc. But first you need to learn the exercises and correct technique. This section includes:

Pre-gym Warm-up
This should be done every time you visit the gym.

Pre- and Post-cardiovascular/aerobic Stretches
These may be done either before or after any aerobic or cardiovascular activity.

Four Cardiovascular Machines
The following machines may be used either for a short warm-up or a longer aerobic session:
The rowing machine
The bike
The treadmill
The elliptical cross trainer

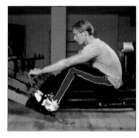
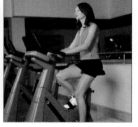
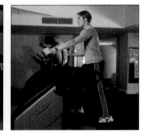

The rowing machine   *The bike*   *The treadmill*   *The elliptical cross trainer*

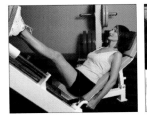

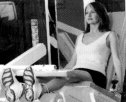

Leg Press	*Hamstring Curls*

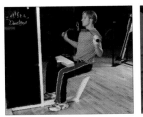

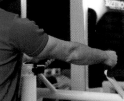

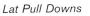

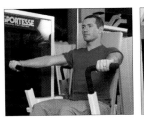

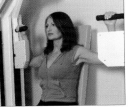

Lat Pull Downs	*Machine Rows*

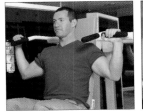

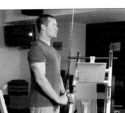

Chest Press	*Pec Deck*

Shoulder Press

Push Downs

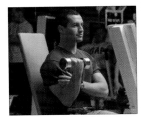

Biceps Curls

Nine Machine Bases

You can then choose which of the nine machine bases you wish to include. For guidance, refer to the Gym Workouts at the end of this section. Each machine base has a relevant stretch to do afterwards.

- Leg Press
- Hamstring Curls
- Lat Pull Downs
- Machine Rows
- Chest Press
- Pec Deck
- Shoulder Press
- Push Downs
- Biceps Curls

Abdominal Exercises

Wind-down

These exercises should be done each time you workout to rebalance the body.

Gym Workouts

To help you plan your sessions at the gym we have given you seven different workouts to do and advice on combining the different elements of your fitness programme.

Warm-up

This short routine is your mental and physical preparation for the activities ahead. The following exercises are designed to remind you how to move correctly.

You can wear gym shoes for these exercises but please note that later in the programme you may need to remove them.

Roll Downs ○ 🚴 🤸

Aim

To release tension in the spine, the shoulders and the upper body. To mobilise the spine, creating flexibility and strength and achieving segmental control. To teach correct use of stabilising abdominals when bending.

Please take advice if you have a back problem (see below), especially disc-related.

You may prefer to do the version of this exercise against the wall – see page 130.

This fabulous exercise can be used during your warm-up or your wind-down with equal effect. It combines stabilising work with the wonderful wheeling motion of the spine. As you roll back up, think of rebuilding the spinal column, stacking each vertebra one on top of another to lengthen out the spine.

Starting Position

- Stand correctly remembering all the directions on page 26. You may leave your shoes on.

Action

1. Breathe in wide and full to prepare, lengthening up. Bend your knees a little.

2. Breathe out, zip up and hollow (stay zipped throughout now), drop your chin onto your chest and allow the weight of your head to make you slowly roll forward, head released, arms hanging, centre strong, knees soft.

3. Breathe in as you hang, really letting your head and arms release.

4. Breathe out, firmly zipped up and hollowed, as you drop your tailbone down, directing your pubic bone forward. Rotate your pelvis backwards as you slowly come up, rolling through the spine, rebuilding the spinal column bone by bone.

5. Repeat six times.

Watchpoints

- You may like to take an extra breath during the exercise. This is fine, but please try to breathe out as you move the spine.

- Make sure that you go down centrally and do not sway over to one side. When you are down, check where your hands are in relation to your feet.
- Do not roll the feet in or out. Keep the weight evenly balanced and try not to lean forward onto the front of your feet or back onto your heels.

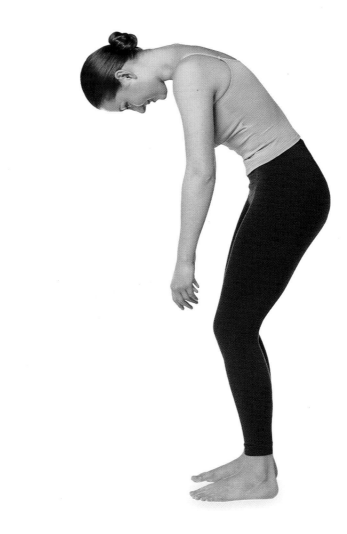

Shoulder Circles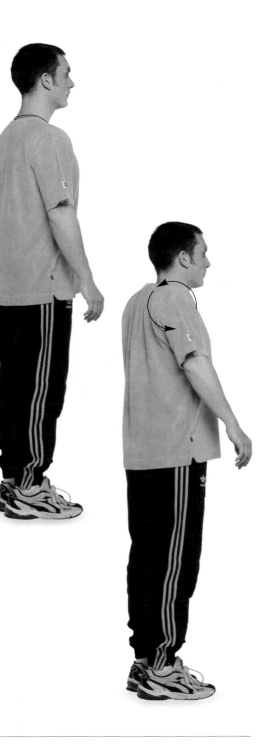

Aim

To mobilise the shoulder area.

This exercise continues our theme of releasing tension and mobilising the upper body. Do not be tempted to do the circles too quickly; the slower and the deeper you make the movement, the more beneficial it is. Done correctly, it should feel like a good massage.

Starting Position

- Stand correctly – see page 26.

Action

1. Breathing normally, continually lengthening up through the spine, draw imaginary circles with your shoulders, rolling them forward, then up towards your ears, back and down into your back before coming forward and around again. Your arms will hang.
2. Repeat ten times but in one direction only, forward and up and then down into the back.

Watchpoints

Take care that you keep your neck long and released.

The Corkscrew ↻ 🚴

Aim

To learn the correct placement and mechanics of the shoulders.

Why is it called the corkscrew? Imagine the type of corkscrew where as the arms are brought down the cork pops up – this is like your head coming up as your arms descend.

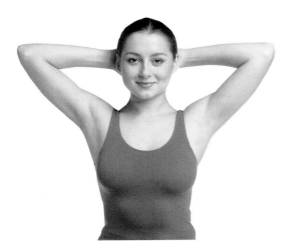

Starting Position

- Stand correctly (page 26), your weight evenly balanced, spine lengthened, gently zipped up and hollowed.

Action

1. Breathe in to prepare and lengthen up through the spine.
2. Breathe out, zip up and hollow (stay zipped now throughout the exercise), and allow your arms to float upwards. Keep the upper shoulders relaxed, think of dropping the shoulder blades down into your back as the arms rise. Clasp your hands lightly behind your head.

3. Breathe in as you shrug your shoulders up to your ears.
4. Breathe out as you drop them down.
5. Breathe in as you gently bring your elbows back a little. Your shoulder blades will come together. You should still be able to see them.
6. Breathe out as you release your hands and slowly bring them down to your sides, opening them wide, engaging the muscle beneath your shoulder blades. As you do so, think of allowing the head, neck and spine to lengthen up as the arms come down. Think of the corkscrew.
7. Repeat five times.

Watchpoints

- Remember not to arch the back as you bring your elbows back.
- As you bring the arms up, remember to keep the shoulder blades down for as long as possible by using the muscles below the shoulder blades.

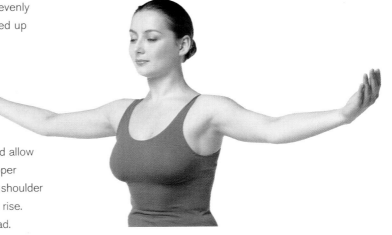

Neck Crescents 🚴

Aim

To release tension gently and safely from the neck and restore a full range of movement to the cervical spine.

Starting Position

- Stand correctly – see page 26.

Action

1. Slowly drop your chin onto your chest, making sure that you do not round your upper back as you do so. Keep your shoulder blades down into your back.

2. Gently roll your chin in a quarter circle to the left, eventually bringing it up to look directly over your left shoulder.

3. Now reverse the action, tracing a semi-circle rolling down and up until you are looking directly over your right shoulder.

4. Repeat six times.

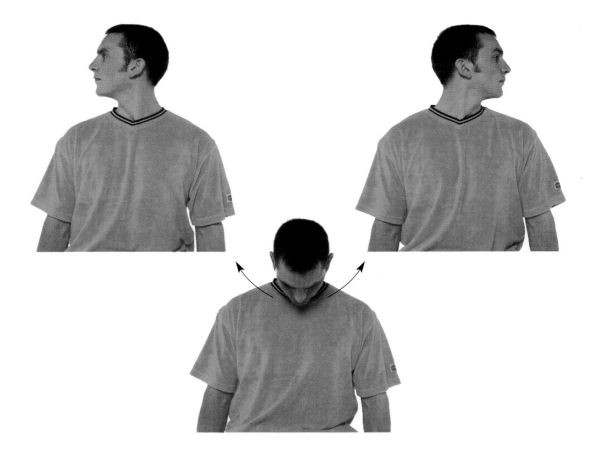

Waist Twists (The Cossack) ↻ 🚴

Aim

To learn how to rotate the spine safely with stability and length.

Starting Position

- Stand correctly – or sit tall on a sturdy chair. You may leave your shoes on.
- Fold your arms so that the top arm is resting lightly on the underneath arm, creating a rectangular shape.
- Your arms should be just above your waist, shoulder blades down into your back, upper shoulder relaxed.

Action

1. Breathe in as you lengthen up through the spine.
2. Breathe out, zip up and hollow and, keeping your pelvis square and facing forward, gently turn your upper body round as far as is comfortable. Your head will turn also. Only turn as far as you can; keep your pelvis square and still.
3. Breathe in as you return to centre.
4. Repeat up to ten times to each side.

Watchpoints

- Do not allow the shoulders to creep up around the ears. Keep the shoulder blades down into the back.
- Try to keep the weight evenly balanced on both feet.
- Do not turn the head too far. It should move naturally, balanced on top of the spine.

- Try not to tilt forward with one shoulder, stay central.
- If you find your pelvis moving, stand in front of a table or the back of a chair with your thighs just touching it – this tells you when you twist the pelvis.

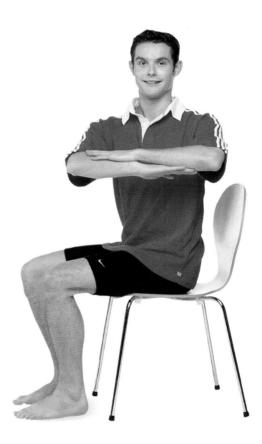

Walking on the Spot plus Calf Stretch 🚴 🤸 ♡

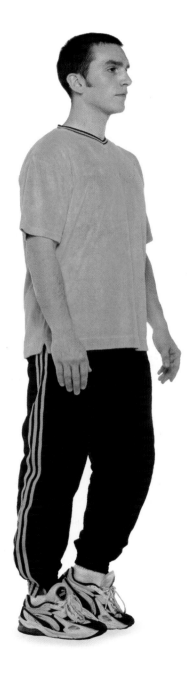

Aim

To warm-up the legs, mobilising the ankle joints, re-affirming good leg alignment and gently stretching the calves. It also starts to get the circulation going.

A simple exercise which can be done anywhere, yet it is deceptively hard to do well. The key is to keep good body alignment throughout. You have three main body weights, your head, your ribcage and your pelvis. Try to keep them balanced centrally on top of each other. When you bend your knees in this exercise, they should bend directly over the second toes. You may have to check this occasionally during the exercise.

Starting Position

- Stand correctly – see page 26. Your feet are hip-width apart.

Action

1. Breathing normally, come up onto the balls of your feet, making sure that your body doesn't pitch forwards. Then drop your left heel back down; your right knee bends over your foot as you do so.
2. Swap legs so that you are in effect walking on the spot. The idea is to keep lengthening upwards, your weight staying centred, your pelvis level and your waist long.

Watchpoints

- Try not to lean forward.
- Do not collapse.
- Try not to wiggle your hips around. Your pelvis stays level and neutral throughout.

Warming-Up and Cardiovascular Work

The following cardiovascular machines are common to most fitness clubs:

- the rowing machine
- the bike
- the treadmill
- the elliptical cross trainer

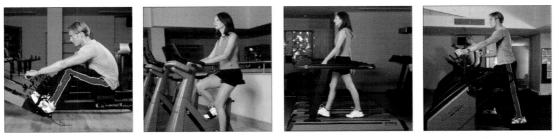

The rowing machine	*The bike*	*The treadmill*	*The elliptical cross trainer*

You can use these machines as part of your warm-up or for more intense cardiovascular training. In either case, the guidelines will apply, but how long you spend exercising and the intensity you choose will obviously differ depending on whether you wish merely to raise your body temperature or build your aerobic strength.

As with all forms of warming-up, the length of time will depend on the temperature of the venue and the outside temperature from where you have just arrived. For instance, if either the room or you are cold spend a little longer on your warm-up. As a general guideline, the time spent warming-up should range from five to ten minutes.

Remember the Six Golden Rules and remind yourself of the general guidelines on aerobic work on page 17.

Gentle Pre- and Post-aerobic Stretches

These five preparatory stretches may be used before you start your aerobic workout or short warm-up on the machines. They may also be used after your cardiovascular activity as a gentle wind-down.

Standing Quadriceps Stretch

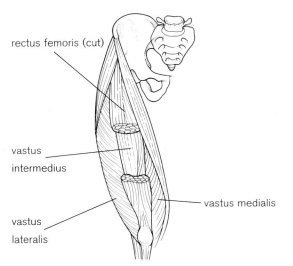

rectus femoris (cut)

vastus intermedius

vastus medialis

vastus lateralis

The quadriceps at the front of your thigh

Aim

To stretch the front of the thighs while maintaining correct body alignment.

Please take advice if you have a knee injury.

Equipment

A scarf (optional). See Watchpoints below.

Starting Position

- Stand alongside the wall placing your left hand on the wall for support and remembering all the directions for standing correctly (page 26).

Action

1. Breathe in to prepare and lengthen up through the spine.
2. Breathe out, zip up and hollow and bend the right knee so that you can clasp the ankle. As you do so, check that you have not arched or bowed your back, it must stay neutral. Imagine there is a small weight attached to your tailbone to help keep the length at the base of the spine.
3. Now gently pull the ankle towards your buttock, keeping the knee still and in line with your other leg. Do not take it too far back. Keep lengthening from the top of your head to your tailbone. Think of also lengthening down through the knee.

4. Hold the stretch, breathing normally, for twenty seconds. Repeat twice on each leg.

Watchpoints

- If you know that you are not flexible or have a knee problem, use a long scarf and place it over the front of your foot to help. Hold the scarf with the same hand and gently bring the foot towards your bottom.
- The most common mistake made with this exercise is to allow the pelvis to shift as the leg bends back. Keep the tailbone lengthening downwards towards the floor and keep the natural curves of the spine, without arching the back.
- Try not to lock the supporting knee joint.
- Keep the shoulder blades down into the back and the neck long.
- Relax. Avoid carrying tension. Keep breathing wide and full.
- Keep both sides of your waist long and your pelvis level.

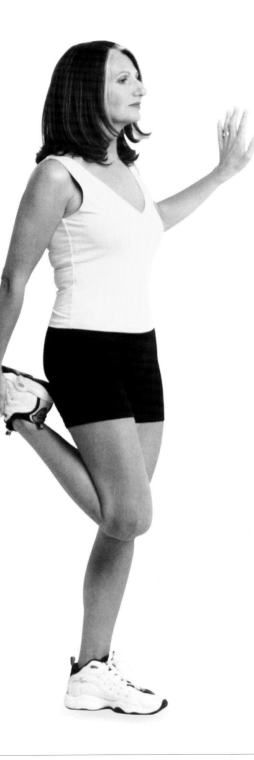

Side-lying Quadriceps Stretch ⬦

Aim

To stretch out the quadricep muscles which run along the front of the thigh and the hip flexors. To lengthen and iron out the front of the body, especially around the front of the hips which can get very tight if you sit all day. To maintain good alignment of the torso, by using the waist muscles and the shoulder stabilisers.

This exercise is an alternative way to stretch the quadriceps and hip flexors and particularly good after cardiovascular work such as the treadmill or bike.

Please take advice if you have a knee injury. You may need to use a scarf to hook over the foot so that there is less pressure on the knee or you may need to leave this exercise out.

Equipment

Scarf and pillow (optional).

Starting Position

- Lie on your side, your head resting on your extended arm (you may like a flat pillow between the head and the arm to keep the neck in line).
- Have the knees curled up at a right angle to your body. Your back should be in a 'straight' line, but with its natural curve.
- Line all your bones up on top of each other – ankle over ankle, knee over knee, hip over hip and shoulder over shoulder.

Action

You must take great care with this exercise not to arch the back. Try to stay in neutral, although we'd rather you tucked under slightly than risk over-hollowing the back.

1. Breathe in wide and full to prepare and lengthen through the spine.

2. Breathe out, zipping up and hollowing, and bend the top knee towards you taking hold of the front of the foot if you can reach it (you may need to use a scarf).

3. Breathe in and check your pelvic position, you should be in neutral. Breathe out, zip up and hollow and gently take the leg back to stretch the front of the thigh. Do not arch the back. Think of the knee lengthening away from the top of the head.

4. Hold the stretch for about twenty seconds, working the waist the whole time, keeping the length in the trunk.

5. After twenty seconds slowly release by bringing the leg back in front of you, zipping up throughout.

6. Repeat three times on each side.

Watchpoints

- Keep the waist long.
- Keep the shoulder blades down into the back and a gap between the arms and the shoulders.
- Do not collapse forward. Keep the upper body open.
- If you cannot reach the foot in the stretch, or the stretch is too great and the knee feels stressed, try using the scarf wrapped over the front of the foot.

Lying Hamstring Stretch

Aim

To stretch the hamstrings while keeping the torso stable, the back anchored and without creating any tension elsewhere in the body. You may keep your shoes on for this if you wish.

Please note: stop immediately if you experience any strange sensations in the legs.

Equipment

A scarf or stretch band.

Starting Position

*   Lie in the Relaxation Position. You may need a cushion for your head.
*   Bring one knee towards your chest.
*   Hold the scarf/stretchband from underneath, your palms towards you. Place the scarf over the sole of one foot.

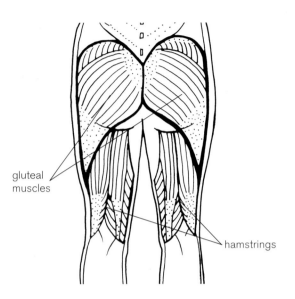

gluteal muscles

hamstrings

The muscles at the back of your leg

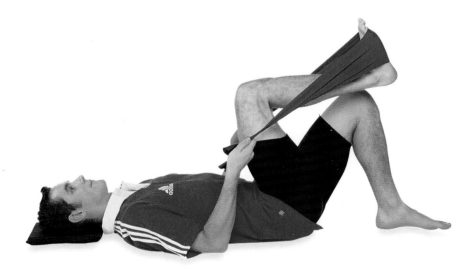

Action

1. Breathe in wide and full to prepare.
2. Breathe out as you zip up and hollow, maintaining neutral pelvis.
3. Slowly straighten the leg into the air, the foot being flexed downwards towards your face. Your tailbone stays down on the floor.
4. Breathing normally now, hold the stretch for the count of twenty to thirty seconds.
5. Relax the leg by gently bending it again.
6. Repeat three times to each leg.

Watchpoints

- Don't allow the pelvis to twist as you straighten the leg – anchoring navel to spine will help you. Keep north to south, east to west.
- Keep your tailbone down as you stretch the leg.
- Check your neck – often the neck shortens and arches back as the hamstrings are stretched. If this happens, place a small flat firm cushion under your head to keep the neck long. Think of softening the neck and breastbone, and of opening the elbows.
- Don't strain – ease the leg out, gently stretching it within your limits.
- Keep the leg in parallel – do not allow it to rotate in or out.

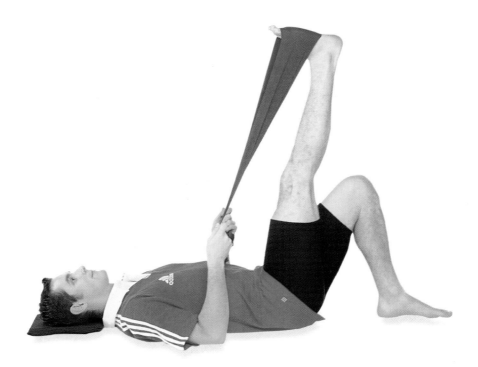

Standing Calf Stretch

Aim

To stretch the calf muscles at the back of the lower leg.

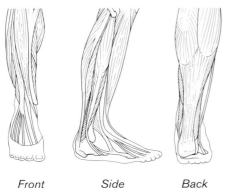

| Front | Side | Back |

Action

1. Stand facing a wall. Place your hands and lower arms (with your elbows bent) against the wall.
2. Gently place the toes of one leg at the base of the wall with the foot pointing forward and the knee bent in line with the ankle.
3. The opposite leg should be placed to the rear. The leg should be straight but not locked at the knee. The toes should be pointing forward and the heel down, creating a stretch in the calf muscles.
4. Keep the weight spread evenly through the feet between the big toe, small toe and heel.
5. Keep your breathing relaxed and even as you hold the stretch for twenty seconds.
6. Release the stretch and then bend back the knee a little to create a stretch deeper in the calf (soleus muscle). Make sure the knee bends directly over the second toe. Hold this deeper stretch for twenty seconds, then release.
7. Repeat twice on each side.

Watchpoints

- Stay zipped up and hollowed throughout the stretch.
- Keep lengthening up through the spine maintaining pelvic and spinal neutral throughout.
- Keep your neck lengthened and released.
- Keep your shoulder blades down into the back.
- Ensure the toes are pointing forward and keep the heels down to enable a more effective and safe stretch.

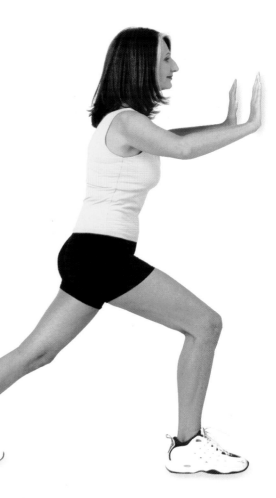

Standing Adductor Stretch

Aim

To stretch the muscles of the inner thigh/groin.

Action

1. Face a mirror if possible.
2. Bend the knee of one leg at a 90° angle to the ankle with the toes pointing in the same direction as the knee.
3. Gradually lengthen the opposite leg away until you feel a gentle stretch in the inner thigh. The toes and knees of this leg should be pointing forward.
4. Keep your shoulders and hips facing forward and place your hands on your hips.
5. Keep your breathing relaxed and even.
6. Hold the stretch for twenty seconds before slowly releasing.

Watchpoints

- Keep zipped up and hollowed throughout.
- Keep lengthening through the spine, maintaining pelvic and spinal neutral.
- Ensure that your head, shoulders and hips stay facing forward.
- The toes and knees should be pointing in the same direction.
- Keep the shoulder blades down into the back and the neck long.

Post-aerobic Stretches

All of the pre-aerobic stretches may be repeated after your cardiovascular workout.

The Machines

The Rowing Machine ♡

The rowing machine provides a perfect warm-up for gym work as it utilises both the upper and lower body. It can also be used as a form of cardiovascular exercise.

There are many brands of rowing machines and the functions vary; just ensure you have the machine set up at a level to suit you and your purpose.

The Rowing Machine as a Warm-up

If you are using the rowing machine as a warm-up, aim to spend five minutes rowing; this should be long enough to raise your body's temperature and warm-up the muscles ready for the machine bases.

The Rowing Machine as a Cardiovascular Workout

If you wish to use the rowing machine as an aerobic workout, you should aim to spend between ten and twenty minutes rowing (ideally work up to 20 minutes for aerobic benefit), depending on your level of fitness. Similarly, alter the resistance to suit your fitness level.

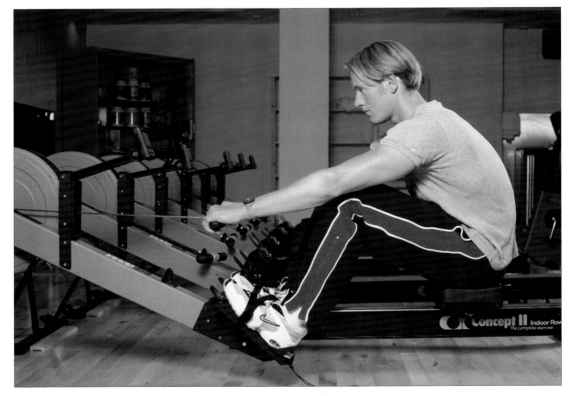

The rowing machine

Guidelines for Using the Rowing Machine

1. Before you begin, set the resistance to a level to suit you goal (warm-up or workout).

2. Remember that your back should remain in good alignment as you move.

3. Pull the bar towards your midriff on the out-breath, zipping up and hollowing.

4. Keep your elbows close to your sides and push through your legs as you pull back.

5. Your shoulders should stay low and your neck long.

6. Breathe in as you return to the Starting Position. Allow the back and arms to stretch at this point.

7. Do not allow your knees to open outside the bar as you return to the Starting Position.

8. Keep your movement smooth and controlled.

How Not To Do It

Common mistakes include:

- Allowing the bar to bounce off the midriff as you pull it towards you.
- Pulling the bar too high or too low at the mid-section of your body.
- Opening the knees on either side of the bar as you return to the Starting Position.
- Leaning back as you pull.
- Shrugging the shoulders and shortening the neck.

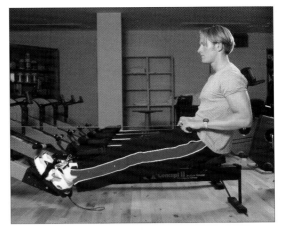

Good technique

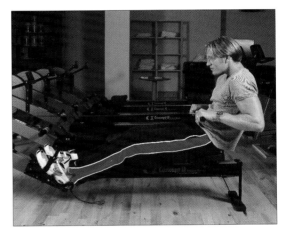

Bad technique

The Bike ♡

The aim of the cycling machine is to improve your heart and lung performance and to work the legs. Most machines are adjustable so that you can increase the resistance of the pedals, simulating cycling uphill. Set the machine at its lowest setting to begin with and then gradually build up your speed and resistance.

The Bike as a Warm-up

Spend approximately five minutes cycling, just enough to raise your body's temperature.

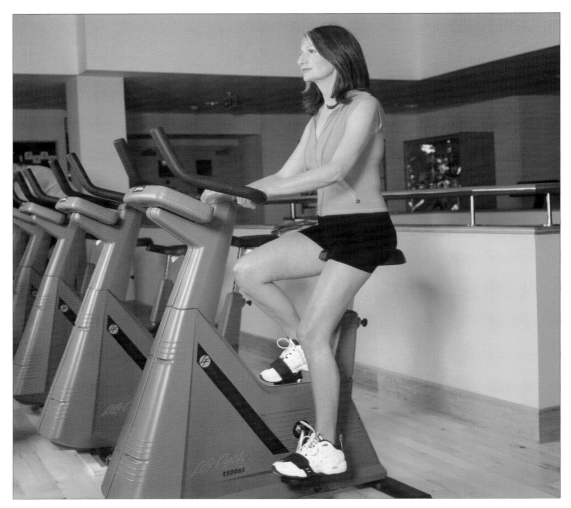

The bike

The Bike as a Cardiovascular Workout

To use the bike as an aerobic workout, increase your cycling time to between ten and ultimately twenty minutes depending on your level of fitness (ideally work up to 20 minutes for aerobic benefit). Alter the resistance accordingly.

Guidelines for Using the Bike

1. Ensure the seat is positioned at a height to suit you. When your foot is at the lowest point on the pedal, your leg should be comfortably stretched but never hyper-extended (locked).
2. Use only enough resistance and speed to raise the body temperature and heart rate.
3. Keep the shoulders relaxed and low. Your neck should be long and the chest open.
4. Your breathing should be steady and relaxed.
5. Pedal evenly, trying to put equal pressure on each leg.

How Not To Do It

Common mistakes include:

- Leaning forward heavily on the handlebars, which will put pressure on the neck and shoulders and you'll lose your alignment.
- Allowing the knees to dip towards the mid-line or fall open, which will result in uneven wear and tear on the knee joints.
- Having the seat too high or too low; both will put strain on the low back and pressure on the discs.

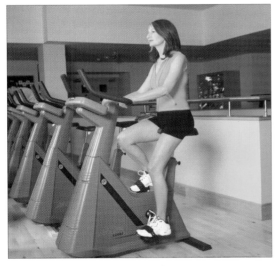

Good technique

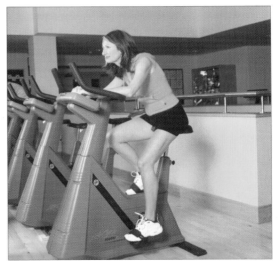

Bad technique

The Treadmill ♡

The treadmill is designed for running or walking. It is ideal to use as a tool for raising the body temperature and heart rate, for a warm-up or as part of a cardio-vascular programme.

Some treadmills have in-built heart-rate monitors (if not try to use your own) and most have a choice of programmes to suit the individual. For a warm-up, we advise you to set the machine at a speed that allows you to walk briskly but comfortably, raising the heart rate and body temperature steadily in preparation for the work ahead. Each of us is built differently so the speed will depend on your stride and on your fitness

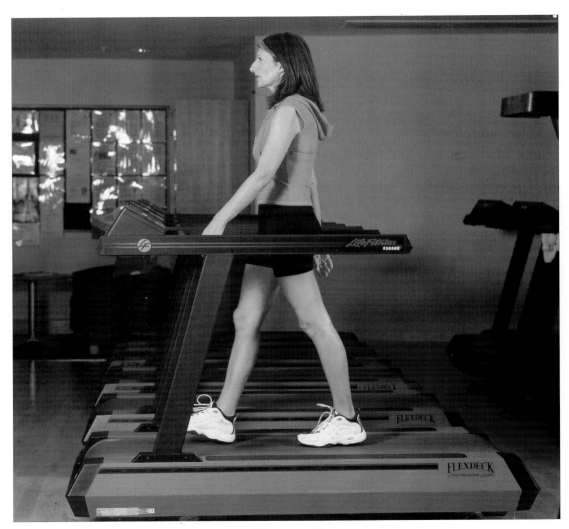

The treadmill

level (generally the lower your cardiovascular fitness the quicker your heart rate will rise, so be careful).

A quality treadmill will also have incline options that allow you to simulate hill walking or running, but for the purpose of warming-up set the gradient at its lowest point and focus on the speed of the machine.

The Treadmill as a Warm-up

Aim to spend just five minutes brisk walking to begin with especially if your fitness level is low. This should be long enough to raise your heart rate. If you have a good level of fitness, you can start to jog.

The Treadmill as a Cardiovascular Workout

Depending on your level of fitness, you can work up to twenty minutes on the treadmill. If your level of fitness is low, start with brisk walking then, as you become fitter, you can jog or run.

Guidelines When Using the Treadmill

1. Walk briskly at a pace that allows you to raise the body temperature steadily.
2. You should walk with a heel-toe action.
3. Relax your shoulders and swing your arms freely as you walk.
4. Your chest should be open and your breathing relaxed.
5. Keep the length in your body, do not hunch.

How Not To Do It

Common mistakes include:

- Walking or running on the toes, instead of in a heel-toe movement.
- Tensing the shoulders and arms. They should be relaxed and moving freely.

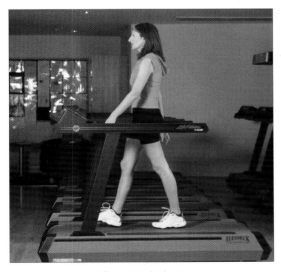

Good technique

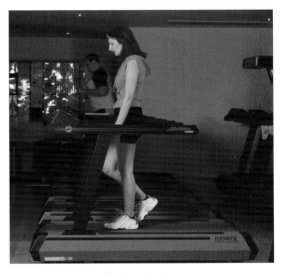

Bad technique

The Elliptical Cross Trainer ♡

The elliptical cross trainer is ideal to use both as a warm-up and as a form of cardiovascular exercise. It has the combined effects of a bike, ski-machine and treadmill. It is low impact and therefore does not affect the knees or lower back.

The Cross Trainer as Warm-up

Set it on a manual programme and spend five minutes to warm-up your muscles.

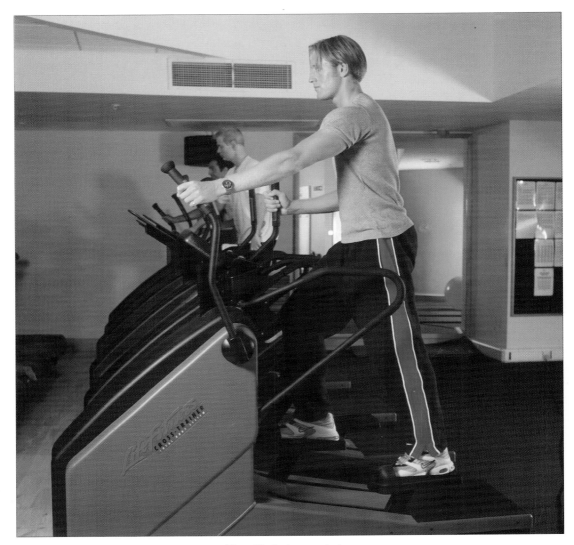

The elliptical cross trainer

The Cross Trainer as Cardiovascular Workout

To begin with, set the machine on a manual programme – there are more advanced programmes that you can opt for when you are fitter. Spend up to twenty minutes exercising, following the guidelines below.

Guidelines When Using an Elliptical Cross Trainer

1. Use a heart-rate monitor if possible.
2. Work at a steady pace monitoring your heart rate on the screen in front of you.
3. Keep the length in your spine, your shoulder blades down into your back and your neck released.
4. Ensure that your feet are pointing forward and close to the top end of the foot panels.
5. Keep your breathing relaxed.

Watchpoints

- Keep the shoulder blades down into the back and the neck long.
- Avoid gripping hard on the hand supports.

How Not To Do It

Common mistakes include:

- Leaning forward and putting pressure on the lower back.
- Losing body alignment by pointing the toes out at an angle instead of facing to the front.
- Leaning back too far.

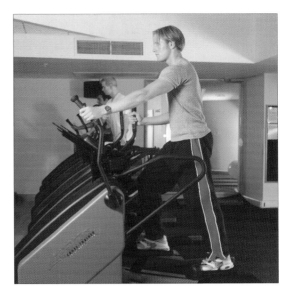

Good technique

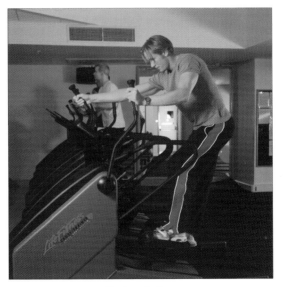

Bad technique

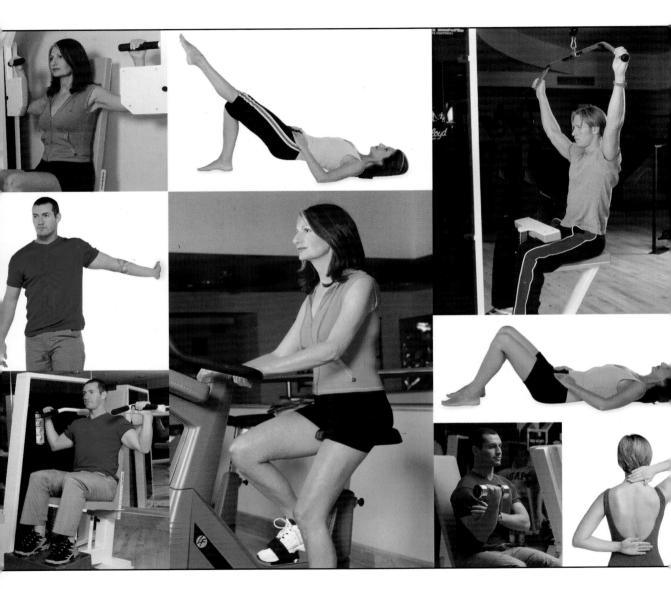

Nine Machine Bases

This part of our workout will show you how to use gym equipment correctly, minimising the risk of injury and maximising the effectiveness of your workouts.

We have taken nine basic weight-training exercises which can be performed in most gyms and fitness centres and which target the main muscle groups of the body.

The majority of these initial exercises are machine-based (Seated Biceps Curls being the exception), so enabling you to execute them using the correct form and technique without the added concern of loss of balance and potential injury. We are asking you to be aware of many things as you train even if you are experienced in the use of weights. Each machine-based exercise is followed by an appropriate stretch or stretches. These stretches may also be done before, in addition to, or after – but not instead of – using the machine.

These exercises are not easy to perform in the way in which we are asking you to do them – remember, it is much easier to perform any exercise incorrectly. However, with the right amount of time and application the benefits will become obvious to you. Remember the Six Golden Rules! Train intelligently. Train safely. Train effectively. Feel and see the benefits.

Please note: we recommend that you use weights no more than two or three times a week to avoid the risk of over-use injuries. Make sure you read the advice given on strength training on pages 7–9. It is very easy to push yourself too hard in the gym by increasing the resistance of the machine or the number of repetitions.

The Leg Press (Machine Base) 🏋

Aim

To strengthen and shape the quadriceps, hamstrings and gluteal muscles.

This is a safe way to target your legs and bottom, due to the back support that a well-designed machine should possess.

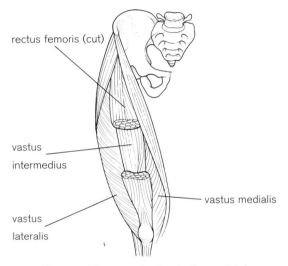

The quadriceps at the front of your thigh

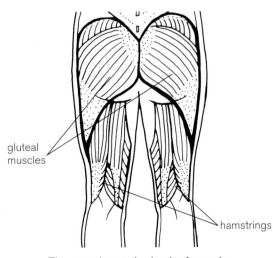

The muscles at the back of your leg

Starting Position

- Set the machine to the correct length for you to enable a full range of motion to take place.
- Start in the straight leg position. Ensure that your feet are hip-width apart in a line with your knees and that there is equal contact on the foot panel between your big toe, small toe and heel, avoiding any rolling in or out of the feet.
- The back of the neck and spine should be in good alignment – place a towel behind your head, if necessary.
- There should be no tension anywhere in the body prior to beginning the exercise.

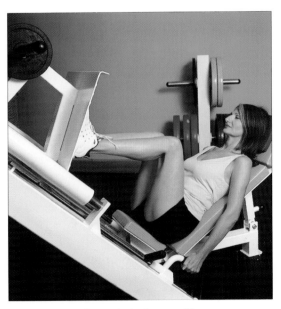

A good starting position

Action

1. Breathe in wide and full to prepare.
2. Breathe out, zip up and hollow (stay zipped throughout now), keeping your pelvis in neutral, lower the weight until your knees are in line with your ankles at 90°.
3. Breathe in, breathe out, zip up and hollow as you push the weight away from you keeping equal pressure through your feet and the centre of your thighs. Avoiding rolling the feet and knees in or out. Keep lengthening up through the spine.
4. Finish your set in the straight leg position.
5. Do eight repetitions.

Watchpoints

- Keep all your movements smooth and controlled.
- Keep the shoulder blades down into the back and your chin tucked in gently. Your upper body must remain relaxed and open. Lengthen the neck to avoid shrugging and unnecessary tension. Relax the chest and front of the shoulders.
- Your arms and hands stay relaxed on equipment handles or at your sides.
- Keep zipping up and hollowing throughout, pelvis neutral, spine lengthened and in neutral, the tailbone lengthening away.
- Although your legs are straight on the upward phase, check that you do not lock them out.
- Double check that your legs only lower to 90° (lower than this can lead to knee injury).

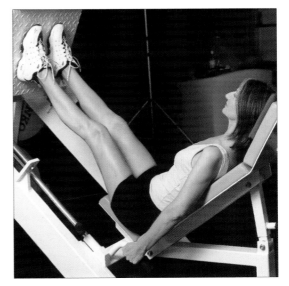

Good technique

How Not To Do It

Wrongly used, this machine could over-extend the back or strain the knee joints.

Common mistakes include:

- Arching the back and lifting your bottom off the seat.
- Allowing the chin to poke forward or tilt backwards, which will strain the neck.
- Allowing the back to move as the legs straighten. If this happens do not fully straighten the legs until your strength and flexibility improve – never fully lock the knees.
- Taking the knees past the line of the hips on the downward phase, thus straining the knees.
- Shrugging the shoulders and shortening the neck.

Follow the Leg Press with the Standing Quadriceps Stretch on pages 54–5.

Hamstring Curls (Machine Base) 🏋️

Aim

To strengthen and shape the hamstring muscles at the back of the upper thigh.

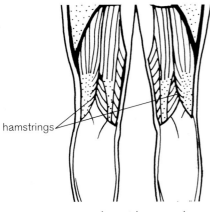

your hamstring muscles

Starting Position

- Set the seat and ankle pads at the correct position for you (the pads should rest just above the Achilles tendons at the back of the heel).
- You may have a pad to secure the front of your thighs; if so, gently hold onto the handles situated on the top of the pad. Alternatively, gently hold onto the handles that should be situated at the sides of the seat.
- The backs of your knees should just clear the end of the seat.
- Your toes, knees and hips should be in line before you start and throughout the exercise.

Action

1. Breathe in wide and full to prepare.
2. Breathe out, zip up and hollow (stay zipped throughout now), keeping your pelvis in neutral and lengthen up through the spine. Now pull the heels towards the machine. Keeping the feet flexed throughout and in a straight line, end the movement when the feet are below the edge of the seat and the hamstring muscles feel fully engaged.
3. Breathe in, still zipped up, as you control the legs back to the Starting Position, lengthening through the hamstrings throughout.
4. Do eight repetitions.

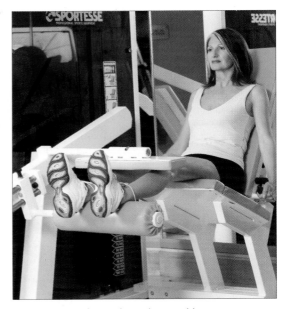

A good starting position

Watchpoints

- Keep all your movements smooth and controlled.
- Keep the shoulder blades down into the back. Your upper body should be relaxed and open. Relax the chest and front of the shoulders. Lengthen the neck to avoid shrugging and unnecessary tension.
- Your arms and hands should stay relaxed on the side or front handles of the equipment.
- Keep zipping up and hollowing throughout, pelvis neutral, spine lengthened and in neutral, the tailbone lengthening away.

How Not to Do It!

Common mistakes include:

- Arching your lower back as you pull the feet towards you. This can happen if the weight is too heavy and/or the feet are pulled too far back.
- Allowing the feet to point (contracting the calves), splay open or turn in.
- Locking the knee joints on return to the Starting Position – control the movement.
- Setting the security pad on the top of the thigh or shin so it allows too much movement.
- Setting the heel pads too high up the lower leg. This lessens the desired tension on the hamstrings.

You can follow the Hamstring Curls with the Hamstring Stretch (pages 58–9).

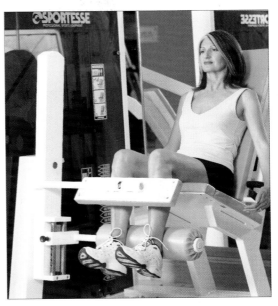

Good technique

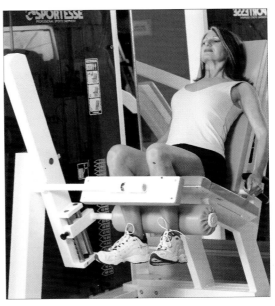

Bad technique

Lat Pull Downs or Wide Pull Downs (Machine Base) 🏋️

Aim

To strengthen and shape the latissimus dorsi muscles.

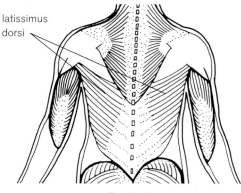

Back view

Starting Position

- Take hold of the wide bar and gently and carefully lower yourself onto the machine seat – if you have a training partner, they can pull the bar down for you while you sit.
- Make sure that you are sitting tall, with neutral spinal and pelvic positions.
- Your feet should be pointing forward and in line with your knees and hips. Your hips should be relaxed and not gripping against the machine's leg rest.
- With this machine, you are sitting holding an overhead crossbar. Initially your upper arms are stretched out to the sides slightly wider and higher than your shoulders.

Action

1. Breathe in wide and full to prepare.
2. Breathe out, zip up and hollow and, maintaining neutral pelvis, pull the bar down to the upper to mid-region of your chest. The elbows are pointing to your hips, the hands in line with and to the sides of the shoulders. The movement should come from your arms and shoulders. Keep the shoulder blades down into the back and the neck lengthened. Focus on isolating the target muscles – the lats.
3. Breathe in as you control moving the bar back to the Starting Position. Keep the shoulder blades down into your back if possible and the

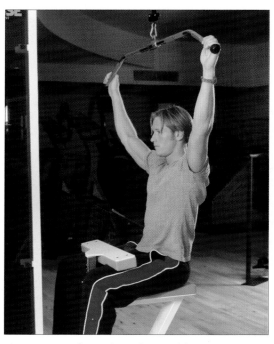

A good starting position

neck long throughout the movement, avoiding any unnecessary shrugging and shortening.

4. Do eight repetitions.

Watchpoints

- Keep the movement smooth and controlled, do not jerk the bar up or down.
- Choose a weight that allows you to perform the correct technique safely and effectively.
- Keep zipping up and hollowing throughout, pelvis neutral, the tailbone lengthening away. It is very easy to arch the lower back during this exercise.
- Keep the shoulder blades down into the back and the neck long throughout.
- Keep your elbows out to the sides as your arms move down. Do not allow them to come forward, or the upper body to close in.
- Avoid gripping the leg rest with your thighs and pushing through the balls of your feet as you pull the bar down. If your centre is strong and your technique efficient you can easily keep this unnecessary tension to a minimum – almost have a feeling of lightness in your legs and feet.

How Not To Do It

Done incorrectly, you can overwork the lats, which will upset the balance of the muscles around your shoulders. Common mistakes include:

- Choosing a weight that is too heavy to control, which means that you lose your core stability.
- Poking your chin forward, risking injury to the neck and shoulders.
- Arching the low back as you pull down – stay in neutral.
- Rounding the low back as you pull down – stay in neutral.
- Avoid over-stretching when the bar is at its highest point; you risk straining your back!
- Leaning back - again, stay in neutral.

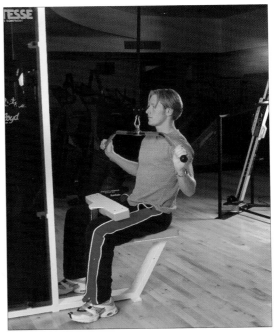

Good technique

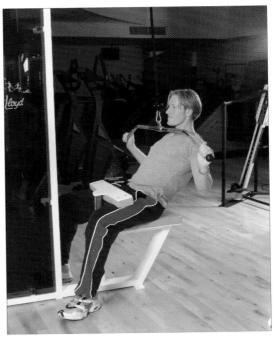

Bad technique

Lat Stretch ⅄

Aim

To stretch the latissimus dorsi gently.

Starting Position

* Sitting at the pull-down machine, gently hold onto the bar in the same way as you did when performing the exercise. Remember that the length of your limbs will dictate how wide this will be.

Action

1. Breathe in wide and full.
2. Breathe out, zip up and hollow, pelvis neutral and tailbone lengthening away.
3. Remain in this Starting Position phase of the lat pull-down exercise, but focus now on lengthening the muscles of the outer back. Do not over-stretch.
4. Hold the stretch for six breaths.

Watchpoints

* Choose enough weight to feel the stretch – no more. The weight should not be lifting you out from the seat. You should only feel a mild tension in the outer back as you stretch the lateral muscles of the back.
* Keep zipping and hollowing throughout, pelvis neutral and tailbone lengthening away.
* Relax, release, keep breathing wide and full.
* Keep the shoulder blades down into the back and the neck long.

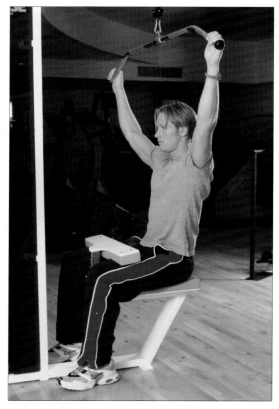

The Lat Stretch

Machine Rows (Machine Base) 🏋️

Aim

To strengthen and shape the muscles of the mid and outer back.

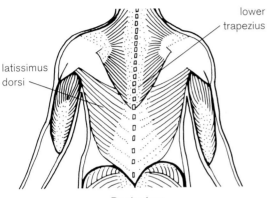

Back view

Action

1. Breathe in wide and full to prepare.
2. Breathe out, zip up and hollow, maintaining neutral pelvis as you start to pull the bars towards you. The movement should end with the bars just in front of your midriff.
3. Breathe in, stay zipped, as you control the weight back down. Try not to let the weights touch as you lower them.
4. Do eight repetitions.

Watchpoints

- Keep the movement smooth and controlled.
- Choose a weight that allows you to perform the correct technique safely and effectively.

Continued ▶

Starting Position

- Sit squarely at the machine.
- Choose the right height for you – your chest and stomach should be resting gently against the padded rest area. The bars of the machine should be at arm's length in front of you.
- Your feet should be facing forward and in line with your knees and hips.
- Check that your spine and pelvis are in neutral.

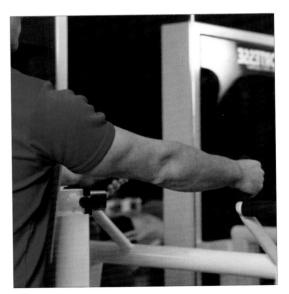

The bars should be at arms length

◄ Continued

- Keep zipping up and hollowing throughout, pelvis neutral, tailbone lengthening away.
- Pull equally with both arms.
- Try to keep your wrists in line. Do not allow them to fold back as you pull.
- Keep the shoulder blades down into the hips and the neck long.

How Not To Do It

Common mistakes include:
- Arching the low back when you pull the weight towards you. This could strain your back.
- Leaning back to assist the pull. This usually happens if the weight is too heavy.

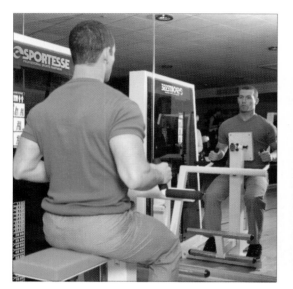

Good technique

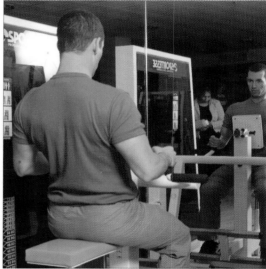

Bad technique

Long Stretch

Aim

To stretch the latissimus dorsi.

Starting Position

- Hold onto the upright structure of the machine gently with one hand — see photo.

Action

1. Breathe in wide and full to prepare.
2. Breathe out, zip up and hollow, maintain neutral pelvis and lengthen up through the spine, walk your feet backwards until the arm is straight and is in line with your shoulder. The knees are bent and the thighs relaxed. Emphasise the stretch by lengthening through the tailbone.
3. Breathe normally now, your opposite hand resting gently above your elbow. The back of your head should be in line with your spine (you can rest your head on the forearm of the supporting arm). Your knees should be bent and your bottom is gently pushed away to encourage the stretch in the outer back.
4. Hold for six breaths. Repeat on other side.

Watchpoints

- Keep zipping up and hollowing throughout, pelvis neutral and tailbone lengthening away.
- Try not to let the pelvis twist off-centre, keep it square. Placing the opposite hand above your elbow should discourage this.
- Keep the shoulder blades down into the back, and the neck long.
- Relax and release any tension in the body. Keep breathing wide and full.

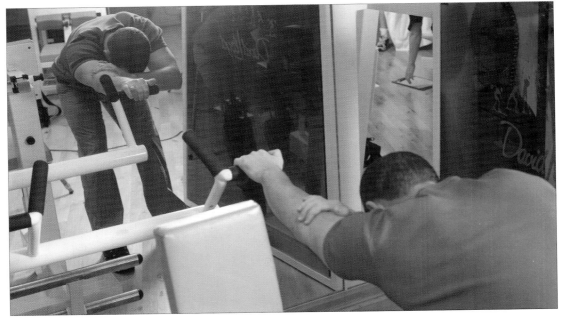

The Long Stretch

Chest Press (Machine Base)

Aim

To strengthen and shape the pectoral muscles.

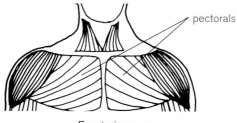

Front view

Action

1. Breathe in wide and full to prepare.
2. Breathe out, zipping up and hollowing, pelvis neutral as you push the hands away from you. Straighten the arms at the end of the movement without locking the elbows. Focus on engaging/contracting the chest muscles.
3. Breathe in, still zipped, as you control the hands back towards the chest.
4. Do eight repetitions.

Starting Position

• Sit in a central position on the machine. Use a mirror as a guide if possible.

• The head should be in line with the spine. Place a towel behind your head if needed.

• Your feet are flat on the floor, in line with the knees and hips. If your feet cannot touch the floor, put them on an exercise step. This will ensure alignment and will protect the lower back.

• Your hands are placed on the bars in front of you with the knuckles pointing forward. The elbows are in line with the hands.

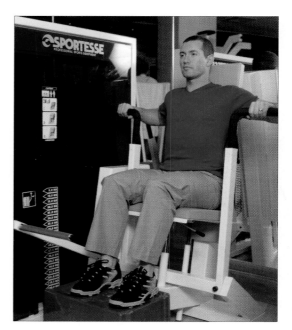

A good starting position

Watchpoints

- Keep the movement smooth and controlled.
- Keep zipping up and hollowing, pelvis neutral, the tailbone lengthening away.
- Beware of the low back arching as you return to the start position. The bars should not come past the line of the chest at any point.
- Ensure that you are not pushing with one side more than the other. You may have to focus on your weaker side a little more to avoid this.
- Make sure that the wrist does not shorten during any point in the exercise.
- Keep the shoulder blades down into the back and the neck long throughout the movement.

How Not To Do It

Once again the dangers of poor technique can lead to back and neck strain. Common mistakes include:

- Shortening the back of your neck and pushing out the chest and ribcage. This can happen if the handles are too far back on the Starting Position (deeper than the line of the chest).
- Arching the low back for the same reason as above, thus straining the back.
- Locking out the elbows.

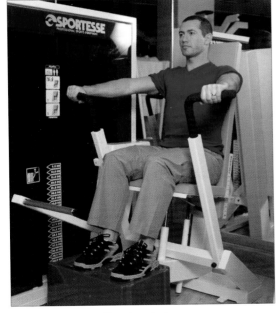

Good technique

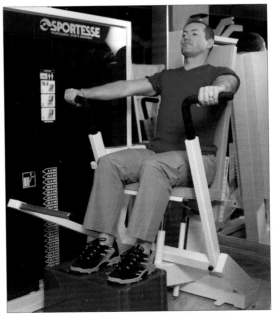

Bad technique

Pec Deck Stretch

Aim

To stretch the pectorals.

Starting Position and Action

1. Sit on the machine and position your body as though you were about to begin the exercise (see above). Lengthen through the spine.
2. Set the push-pads in a position that allows you to feel a *very* gentle stretch across the chest.
3. Zip up and hollow throughout, maintaining your neutral pelvis.
4. Hold the stretch for six breaths.

Watchpoints

- Do not over-stretch. Choose enough weight to feel the stretch and nothing more! You should feel only a mild stretch across the chest. Any more and you risk damage to the shoulder joint.
- Relax, releasing any tension.
- Keep the shoulder blades down into the back, and the neck long.

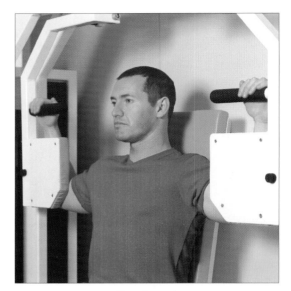

Pec Stretch

Pec Deck (Machine Base)

Aim

To strengthen and shape the pectoral/chest muscles, while stabilising the shoulder blades.

Starting Position

Try to choose a machine opposite a mirror so you can see if your posture is correct.

- Sit centrally on the machine.
- Position your feet flat on the floor, or on an exercise step if height is a problem, in line with your knees and hips.
- The back of your head should be in line with your spine. Place a towel behind your head, if needed.
- Ensure that your arms are placed at an angle of 90°. The palms of your hands and inside lower arms are flat up against the pads to the side of you. The backs of the upper arms are in line with your armpits.

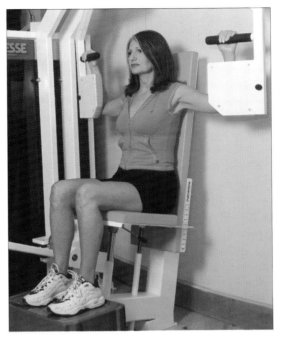

Pec Dec – seating position

Action

1. Breathe in wide and full to prepare.
2. Breathe out, zip up and hollow, maintaining neutral pelvis and lengthening the tailbone away. Push the pads with equal pressure towards the mid-line of the body. Keep the shoulder blades down into the hips and the neck long.
3. End the movement when the pads are at the mid-line of the body. Try not to let them touch.
4. Breathe in, still zipped, as you return under control to the Starting Position.
5. Try not to let the pads touch as you close them in.
6. Do eight repetitions.

Watchpoints

- Choose a weight that allows you to perform the correct technique safely and effectively.
- Keep your movements smooth and controlled.
- Keep zipping up and hollowing throughout, pelvis neutral and the tailbone lengthening away.
- Ensure that you are working each side equally.
- Keep the shoulder blades down into the back and the neck long.

Continued ▶

How Not To Do It

Common mistakes include:

- Arching the low back, pushing the chest and ribcage out and shortening the neck. This can be the result of a Starting Position that takes the arms beyond the line of the chest and shoulders. You risk causing injury to the pectoral area, especially if you lack flexibility there. Your shoulder blades must stay down your back.

- Losing scapular stability. The most common problem is if your seat is set too low or too high. When you do this, you not only invite injury but you are also not using the pectoral muscles efficiently.
- Allowing the pads to touch. The pads should come close together but not touch in the centre in the push phase of the exercise – this contact would result in a momentary loss of tension at a crucial time.

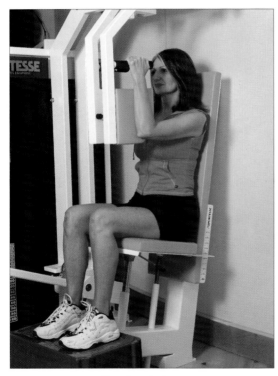

Good technique

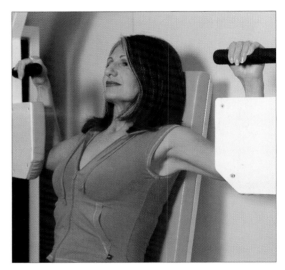

Bad technique

Pec Stretch: Through the Doorway

You can either repeat the stretch on page 84 or try this one!

Aim
To stretch the pectoral muscles of the chest.

Action
1. To stretch the right pectoral muscle, place the hand and back of the lower arm flat against the frame of a doorway or the upright of a weights machine. The elbow should be at a 90° angle, in line with the hand and the armpit. Keep your shoulder blades down into your back.
2. Keeping good spinal and pelvic alignment, bring the right leg forward and the outer hip in line with the door frame. The opposite leg remains at the rear. Ensure that the toes, knees and hips are pointing forward.
3. You should feel a gentle stretch, hold this for about thirty seconds, breathing normally, before stretching the left side.

Watchpoints
- The stretch should be very gentle otherwise you risk injury to the shoulder joint.
- The opposite arm stays relaxed, shoulder blade down into the back.
- Keep the breathing relaxed.
- Keep zipped up and hollowed, pelvis neutral and spine lengthened throughout.
- Ensure that the toes, knees and hips are always pointing forward and that the spine does not twist.
- Keep the shoulder blades down into the back and the neck lengthened and released.

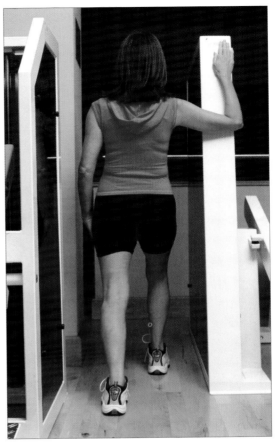

Pec Stretch: Through the Doorway

Shoulder Press (Machine Base) ♟

This is probably one of the hardest machine bases. It is very easy to overwork the upper shoulder muscles. We recommend that you only include this machine base if you are very strong.

Aim

To strengthen and shape the muscles around the shoulder joint (deltoids).

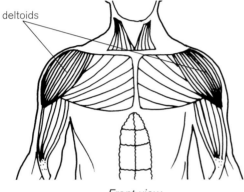

Front view

Starting Position

* Your feet should be flat on the floor, in line with the knees and hips.
* Check that you have your spine in neutral and that the back of your head is in line with the spine. Place a towel behind your head, if needed.
* The hands are placed on the grips with the knuckles pointing towards the ceiling. The elbows should be in line below the hands.

Action

1. Breathe in wide and full to prepare.
2. Breathe out, zip up and hollow, maintaining your pelvis in neutral, as you push the arms up above until you reach full extension, keeping the shoulder blades down into the back and keeping the neck long. Focus on engaging the shoulder muscles at the top end of the movement.
3. Breathe in, still zipped, as you control the descent towards the Starting Position safely.
4. Do five repetitions only.

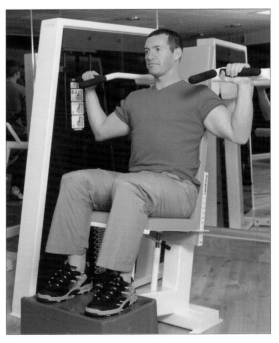

Shoulder Press – seating position

Watchpoints

- Choose a weight that will allow you to perform the correct technique safely and effectively.
- Keep zipping and hollowing throughout, pelvis neutral and the tailbone lengthening away.
- Beware of the lower back arching as you push the bar up. Following the above points will help you to avoid this.
- Ensure that you are not pushing with one side more than the other. You may have to focus on your weaker side a little more to avoid this.
- Keep the shoulder blades down into your back and the neck long throughout the movement.

How Not To Do It

Common mistakes include:

- Arching the low back and losing core stability, which can also cause unnecessary tension in the legs as you push through them to assist the lift.
- Losing scapular stability, pushing through the ribs and shortening the neck.

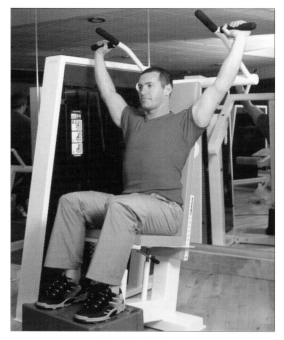

Good technique

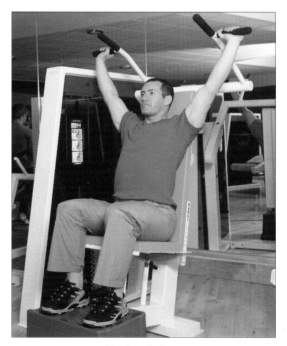

Bad technique

Shoulder Stretch

Aim

To stretch the deltoids, latissimus dorsi and teres major.

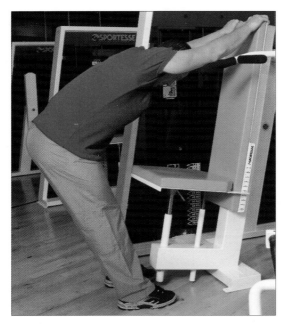

Shoulder Stretch

Starting Position

- Place your hands on the bars of the machine, palms down.
- Walk your feet back until your arms are straight. Try not to lock your elbows out.
- Both feet should be pointing forward. The knees are bent and the thighs relaxed.

Action

1. Breathe in wide and full to prepare.
2. Breathe out, zip up and hollow, maintaining neutral pelvis, and lengthen the tailbone away as you push the bottom away gently. Keep the back of the head in line with your spine.
3. Breathe normally as you focus on stretching the shoulders by lengthening through the tailbone.
4. Hold the stretch for six breaths.

Watchpoints

- Keep zipping up and hollowing throughout, neutral pelvis and tailbone lengthening away.
- Use the breathing to allow any tension to release.
- Keep the shoulder blades down into the back, and the neck long.

Triceps Push Downs (Machine Base)

Aim

To strengthen and shape the triceps muscles at the back of the upper arm, while stabilising the shoulder blades.

Starting Position

- Stand facing the machine with your feet facing forward, in line with your knees and hips.
- Place your hands, palms down, on the bar — preferably a curved bar to protect the wrists.
- Your elbows should be close to your sides, so you may have to adjust your body position in relation to the machine.

Action

1. Breathe in wide and full to prepare.
2. Breathe out, zip up and hollow, maintaining a neutral pelvis as you push the bar towards the floor. Keep the shoulder blades released to the hips as you make the movement. End the push down when the arm is straightened without locking the elbows. Focus on engaging the triceps at the back of your arm at the end of the movement.

3. Breathe in, still zipped, as you control the bar upwards until it is level with your chest. Keep the shoulder blades down into your back to avoid the shoulders lifting.
4. Do eight repetitions.

Continued ▶

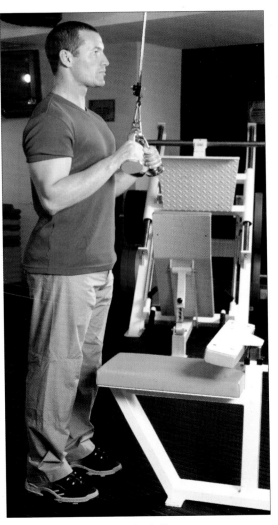

Triceps Push Down

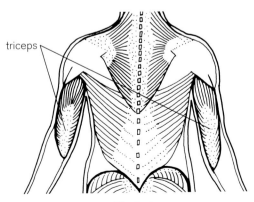

triceps

Back view

◀ Continued

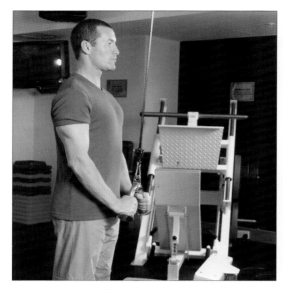

Good technique

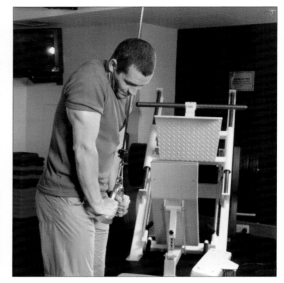

Bad technique

Watchpoints

- Choose a weight that will allow you to perform the correct technique safely and effectively.
- Avoid rocking forwards and backwards. Distribute your weight evenly between your big toe, small toe and heel. The thighs are relaxed with the knee joints slightly open. Balance is the key here. The movement is very small, but the stability required to allow it to be performed correctly must be exact.
- On the downward phase, do lean forward over the bar to assist the contraction. Stay zipped up and hollowed, in neutral and with the shoulders engaged down towards the hips. This will help you to isolate the triceps and achieve the desired contraction. The only tension felt in the body should be in the targeted triceps muscles and the transverse abdominis muscles of the stomach as you zip up and hollow.
- During the return phase observe the points above. If you do not, your shoulders will elevate and your neck will shorten, making you lose your alignment, causing unnecessary tension. Keep looking forward with the neck released.
- Ensure that you are pushing down equally with both arms. Your stronger side may try to take over, especially when fatigue sets in.

How Not To Do It

Common mistakes include:

- Lifting the shoulders, shortening the neck and allowing the arms to rise with the weight. This will happen when you lose core and scapular stability and the shoulders end up doing the work as the weight is pushed down.
- Rounding the upper back for the same reasons. The front of the shoulders (deltoids) roll forward incorrectly assisting the movement and preventing the isolation of the triceps.

Triceps Stretch

Aim
To stretch the triceps at the back of the upper arm. To open the upper body, enjoying lateral breathing.

Equipment
A scarf or stretch band (optional).

Starting Position
- Sit or stand with your pelvis in neutral. Place one hand on the back of your head, at the top of your spine, the other hand at the base of the spine. Keep a sense of openness in the front of your body, but do not allow the back to arch.

Action
1. Breathe in to prepare and lengthen up through the spine.
2. Breathe out, zip up and hollow and start tracing the spine with your fingers until both hands meet. Quite probably they will not be able to meet – please do not force them – use the scarf or stretch bend to help bring them together. Do not allow your upper back to arch.
3. Take two deep breaths, keeping your head central and your ribs wide.
4. Breathe out, zip up and hollow and slowly trace your spine as you take your arms back to the Starting Position.
5. Repeat three times on each side. It is common for one side to be harder than the other.

Watchpoints
- Do not allow the head to twist or tilt to one side.
- Do not allow the back to arch.
- Keep lengthening upwards.

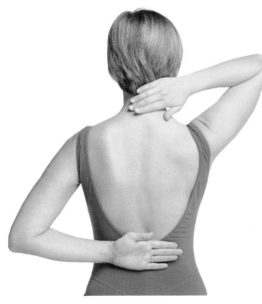
Starting position

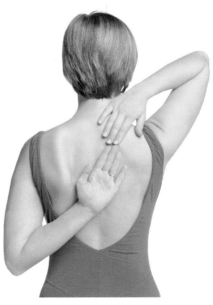
Full position

Seaed Biceps Curls (Dumb-bells)

Aim

To strengthen and shape the biceps muscles at the front of the upper arm while stabilising the shoulder blades.

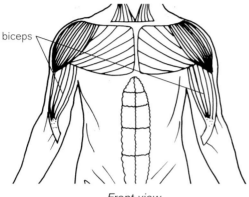

biceps

Front view

Starting Position

- Preferably choose a bench opposite a mirror to study your form.
- Your head should be in line with your spine.
- Place your feet flat on the floor with the toes pointing forward. Feet, knees and hips should be in alignment.
- Hold the weight in one hand, palm facing your thigh. Move your other hand across and lightly hold your arm just above the elbow.

Action

1. Breathe in wide and full to prepare.
2. Breathe out, zip up and hollow, maintaining the pelvis in neutral and lengthening up through the spine. As you raise the arm, gently and slowly rotate your forearm inwards and outwards, keeping the elbow quite still and close into your side. Your hand should finish just in front of your shoulder.
3. Breathe in, still zipped, as you begin to lower the weight under control.
4. Do eight repetitions with each arm.

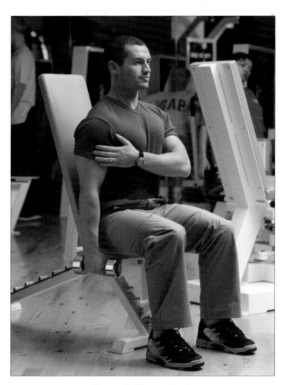

Seated Bicep Curls

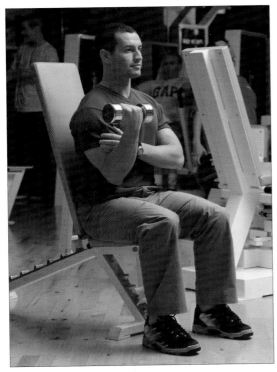

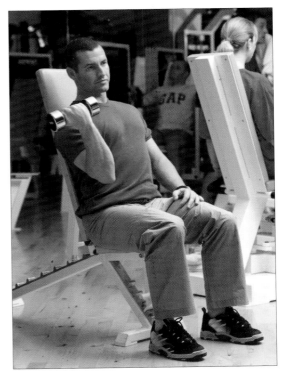

Good technique *Bad technique*

Watchpoints

- Choose a weight that will allow you to perform the correct technique safely and effectively.
- Keep zipping up and hollowing throughout, pelvis neutral and tailbone lengthening away.
- Try not to push through your feet or arch your back to assist the lift.
- Keep your shoulder blades down into the back, keep the neck long and your upper body open.
- Your elbows should be close to your sides to avoid excessive movement and to isolate the biceps.
- Try not to allow your wrists to go floppy.

How Not To Do It

Common mistakes include

- Rocking into the back, thus swinging the weight to complete the lift.
- Losing core and scapular stability as the shoulder dips down and to the side in an attempt to lift the weight. This often occurs when a weight is too heavy to perform the correct technique.
- Leaning backwards and arching the back, shortening the neck. Again, this usually happens when an unsuitable weight has been used.

Reverse Palm Stretch

Aim
To stretch the biceps and pectoral muscles.

Starting Position
*   Place the palm of your hand flat against a wall.

Action
1. Keeping the hand on the wall and the arm straight, breathe in wide and full. As you breathe out, zip up and hollow and slowly turn the rest of the body until you begin to feel the stretch running from the front of the lower arm along the biceps and into the pectoral area.
2. Breathe normally, stay zipped, as you hold the stretch for about six breaths before slowly releasing the stretch.
3. Repeat twice on each side.

Watchpoints
*   Enter into this stretch very gently and slowly. It is a very effective and deep stretch.
*   Keep zipping and hollowing, pelvis neutral and lengthening through the tailbone.
*   Use the breath to help release tension from the body.
*   Keep the shoulder blades down into the back, and the neck long.

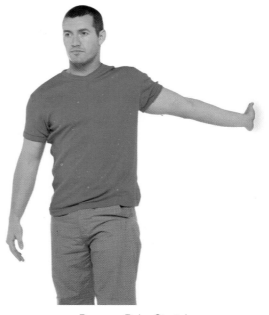

Reverse Palm Stretch

The Abdominals

This next section, which can be done in the gym or at home, concentrates on strengthening the abdominals. You must use a mat and be sure that you stay warm. You will need to remove your shoes for the Single Leg Stretch and the Oblique Leg Stretches. The exercises are progressive, only move on to the next one when you find the current one easy. Proper muscle recruitment is essential, so take your time and work with control.

You have four types of abdominal muscles. Starting from the outer layer, the most superficial is the 'six-pack', the rectus abdominis.

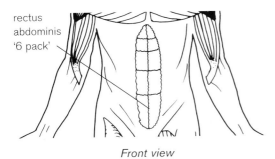

rectus
abdominis
'6 pack'

Front view

This muscle looks superb, but you need to take care that it does not become overdominant. The basic stability exercises in the Girdle of Strength section (page 000) will ensure that you have the necessary inner strength to support a washboard stomach!

Underneath the 'six-pack' you have your external and internal obliques.

These muscles wrap around the waist and are active in twisting and turning movements.

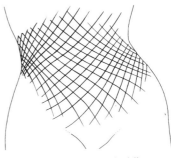

External and internal obliques

And, of course, last but not least, we have the inner core, tranversus abdominis, the importance of which we have already emphasised.

It is only when you have learned how to engage tranversus abdominis, that you will see a real improvement in your rectus abdominis and obliques.

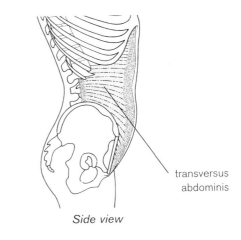

transversus
abdominis

Side view

Curl Ups and Obliques ↻

Aim

To strengthen the abdominals, engaging them in the correct order and with the trunk in perfect alignment. To achieve a flat stomach – well, we all want one!

Please note: avoid this exercise if you have neck problems.

Starting Position

- Lie in the Relaxation Position.
- Gently release your neck by rolling the head slowly from side to side.
- Place one hand behind your head, the other on your lower abdomen – this is to check that your stomach does not pop up. Your pelvis is in its neutral position.

Action

1. Breathe in wide and full to prepare.
2. Breathe out, zip up and hollow, soften your breastbone, tuck your chin in a little as if holding a ripe peach (see page 27) and curl up, breaking from the breastbone.
3. Your stomach must not pop up. Keep the length and width in the front of the pelvis, and the tailbone down on the floor lengthening away. Do not tuck the pelvis or pull on the neck!
5. Breathe in and slowly curl back down.
6. Repeat ten times (change hands after five).

Watchpoints

- Try not to grip around the hips.
- Stay in neutral, tailbone down on the floor and lengthening away. The front of the body keeps its length. A useful image is that there is a strip of sticky tape along the front of the body which should not wrinkle!
- You can take an extra breath while curled up when you are strong enough.

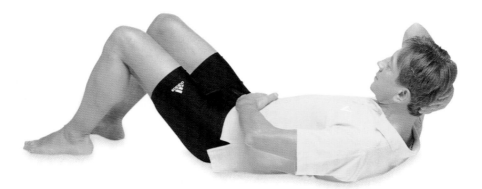

Curl Ups and Obliques

Oblique Curl Ups ↻

Aim

To work the obliques.

Please note: avoid this exercise if you have neck problems.

Starting Position

- As for the previous exercise, only place both hands behind your head, the elbows staying open and just in front of your ears.

Action

1. Breathe in wide and full to prepare.
2. Breathe out, zip up and hollow and bring your left shoulder across towards your right knee. The elbow stays back as it is the shoulder that moves forward. Your stomach must stay hollow, the pelvis stable.
3. Breathe in and lower.
4. Repeat five times to each side.

Watchpoints

- As above, making sure that the pelvis stays square and stable.
- Keep the upper body open.
- Keep the neck released.

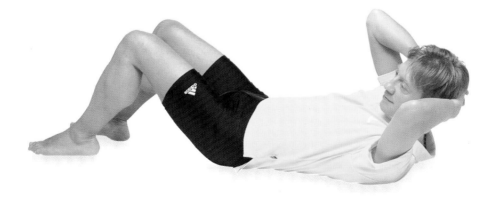

Oblique Curl Ups

Single Leg Stretch (Levels One and Two) 🚴 🤸 C ♡

You will have to remove your shoes for these exercises.

Aim

This is a classical Pilates exercise which is best taught in simple stages. It challenges both the abdominals and your co-ordination. Notice how it combines nearly all the elements of our fitness programme.

Level One

Starting Position

- Lie in the Relaxation Position (page 24), pelvis neutral.

Action

1. Breathe in wide and full to prepare.
2. Breathe out, zipping up and hollowing, and fold one knee at a time on to your chest.

3. Breathe in and take hold of your left leg under the thigh with both hands. Keep your elbows open and your breastbone soft. Your shoulder blades stay down into your back. Neck released.
4. Breathe out, zip up and hollow and slowly straighten the right leg straight up into the air. Try to get approximately a 90° degree angle to the body. Keep your back anchored into the floor.
5. Breathe in and bend the knee back in.
6. Take hold of your right thigh with both hands and repeat the movement with the opposite leg.
7. Repeat ten times with each leg. Do not allow the leg to fall away from you, your back must stay anchored to the floor. When this becomes easy – and only then – you may try the more advanced version below.

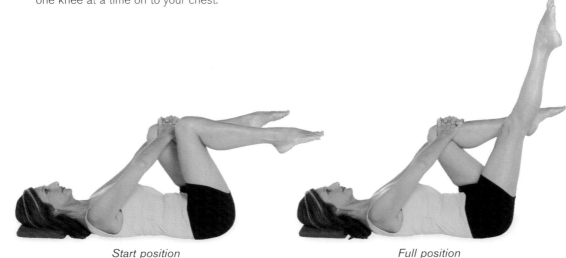

Start position   *Full position*

Level Two

This has to be the best abdominal exercise there is!

Starting Position

- Lie in the Relaxation Position.

Action

1. Breathe in to prepare.
2. Breathe out, zip up and hollow and fold your knees up onto your chest one at a time. The toes just touching, but not the heels. Keep your feet softly pointed. Place the left hand on the outside of the left ankle, the right hand on the inside of the left knee.
3. Breathe in, check that your elbows are open to enable the chest to expand fully. Your shoulder blades are down into your back.
4. Breathe out, zip up and hollow, soften your breastbone and curl the upper body off the floor.
5. Breathe in wide and full.
6. Breathe out and, zipping up and hollowing, slowly stretch your right leg away in parallel, so that it is at an angle of 45° to the floor. The toes are softly pointed.
7. Breathe in wide and full, as you begin to bend the leg back onto your chest, bringing it back into your shoulder.
8. Change hands so that your right hand is now on the outside of your right leg, your left hand on the inside of your right knee.
9. Breathe out and, still zipping up and hollowing, stretch the left leg away in parallel. Do not take it too close to the floor.
10. Breathe in as the leg returns.
11. Repeat ten stretches with each leg, making sure that you have a strong centre throughout and that your shoulder blades stay down into your back, your elbows open.

Watchpoints

- Keep zipping up and hollowing throughout and do not allow the back to arch, the pelvis stays neutral.
- Keep your neck released and the upper body open, shoulder blades down.
- Make sure that you keep the length on both sides of your waist, do not allow one side to shorten.

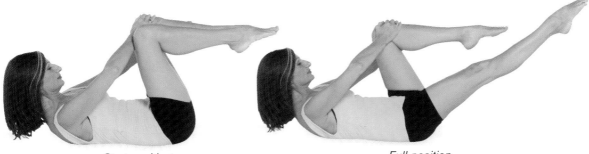

Start position   *Full position*

Oblique Single Leg Stretch or Criss-Cross 🚴 🤸 ↻ ♡

Aim

To work the abdominals, especially the obliques, while challenging co-ordination and core stability.

A powerful exercise that hits the spot. You'll need strong abdominals to do this one correctly.

Starting Position

• Lie on your back, draw your knees up onto your chest, the toes just touching – but not the heels. Keep your feet softly pointed.

• Clasp your hands behind your head. The elbows stay open.

Action

1. Breathe in wide and full to prepare.
2. Breathe out, zip up and hollow as you curl up, softening the breastbone and taking the left shoulder towards your right knee. The upper body stays open, the elbows in line. At the same time straighten the left leg, extending it in parallel at an angle of about 45° to the floor.

3. Breathe out, still zipped up and hollowed, and curl the right shoulder towards the left bent knee, extending the left leg away.

4. Repeat ten times to each side.

Watchpoints

• Make sure that the shoulder, not the elbow, comes across towards the bent knee.

• Keep the elbows in line, do not allow them to come forward. It is your shoulder that is directed towards the knee. In this way, the upper body stays open.

• Stay in neutral please.

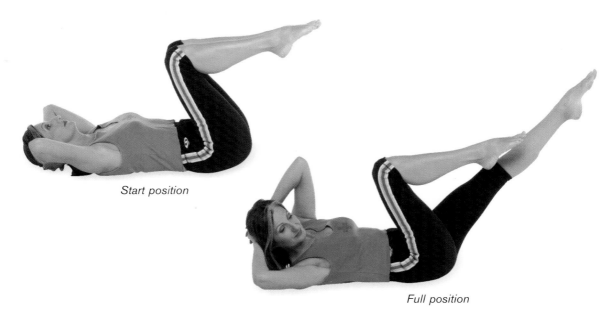

Start position

Full position

The Wind-Down

Your cool-down or wind-down is a vital part of your workout and crucial to maintaining the balance of your body and preventing any feeling of soreness the next day. The exercises have been carefully chosen to complement the work you have been doing in the gym. They take you through movements targeting muscle groups that you may not have used in the main programme. They will also balance the body and help you relax before you rejoin the real world! Shoes off for the wind-down please.

There are six exercises in this section.

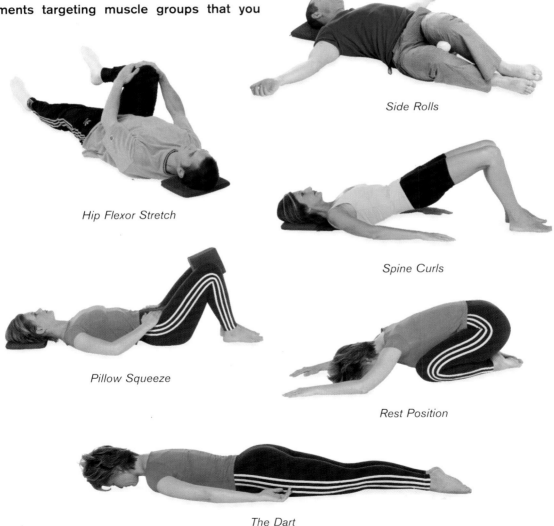

Side Rolls

Hip Flexor Stretch

Spine Curls

Pillow Squeeze

Rest Position

The Dart

Side Rolls C 丫

Aim

To achieve rotation of the spine with stability. To work the obliques (the waist).

Starting Position

*   Lie in the Relaxation Position, have your feet together, in parallel (line up your bunions), and hip-width apart.
*   Place a tennis ball between the knees; this is to help you maintain good pelvic alignment.
*   Place your arms out to the side in line with your shoulders.
*   Allow the floor to support you. Allow your body to widen and lengthen.

Action

1. Breathe in wide and full to prepare.
2. Breathe out, zip up and hollow and roll your head in one direction, your knees in the other. Only roll a little way to start with – you can go further each time if it is comfortable. Keep your opposite shoulder down on the floor.
3. Breathe in, still zipping.
4. Breathe out, use your strong centre to bring the knees back to the Starting Position, the head as well.
5. Repeat eight times in each direction. Think of rolling each part of your back off the floor in sequence and then returning the back of the ribcage, the waist, the small of your back and the buttock to the floor.

Watchpoints

*   Keep the pelvis in neutral, taking care that you do not allow it to arch.
*   Keep working those abdominals. Do not simply allow the weight of the legs to pull you.
*   Try not to let the knees roll apart, the tennis ball should help you avoid this.

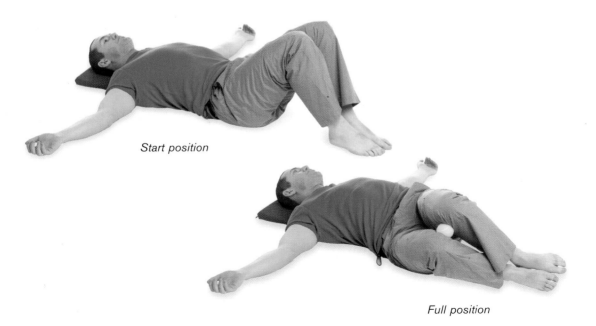

Start position

Full position

Hip Flexor Stretch

Aim

To lengthen the hip flexors gently.

If you sit all day, it is likely that your hip-flexor muscles will shorten. If they do, this will affect the angle of your pelvis, pulling anteriorly.

Starting Position

* Lie in the Relaxation Position.

Action

1. Breathe in wide and full to prepare.
2. Breathe out, zip up and hollow. Keeping that sense of hollowness in the pelvis, hinge the right knee up to your chest, dropping the thigh bone down into the hip joint.
3. Breathe in, as you clasp the right leg below the knee or lower part of the thigh. If you have any knee problems, clasp the leg under the thigh rather than below the knee so that the joint is not compressed.
4. Breathe out, still zipping, and stretch the left leg along the floor. Your lower back should remain in neutral. If it arches, bend the left knee back up again a little.
5. Hold this stretch for five breaths.
6. Breathe in as you slide the leg back.
7. Breathe out, zip up and hollow, as you lower the right bent leg to the floor, keeping the abdominals engaged.
8. Repeat twice on each side, keeping your shoulders relaxed and down.

Watchpoints

* Check the position of the upper body, elbows open, breastbone soft, shoulder blades down into the back, neck released.
* Are you in neutral?
* Keep the stretched leg in contact with the floor.

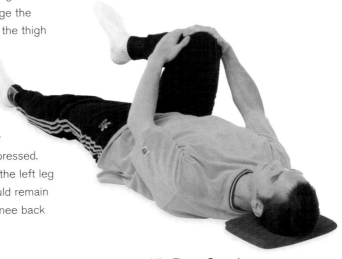

Hip Flexor Stretch

Spine Curls 🚲 C ⅄

Aim

To learn segmental control of the spine at an inter-vertebral level. This is the ability to wheel the spine, vertebra by vertebra, promoting flexibility and stability throughout its length. Joseph Pilates referred to this way of moving as 'using the spine like a wheel'.

In a healthy back all the different segments of the spine work together to create the desired movement, each vertebra contributing to that movement – a bit like a bicycle chain. When one level is locked, the chain is upset. What often happens is that the levels above and below the locked area become over-flexible to compensate for the area that will not move – you can be hypo-mobile (not enough movement) in one area and hyper-mobile (too much movement) above and/or below. This puts enormous strain on the back.

Starting Position

- Lie in the Relaxation Position, your feet about twenty centimetres from your buttocks, hip-width apart and in parallel. Plant the feet firmly onto the floor.
- If it is comfortable, take your arms behind your head and rest them on the floor, keeping them wider than shoulder-width, relaxed and open – your upper back must not be arched. Otherwise, leave your arms down by your sides, palms down.

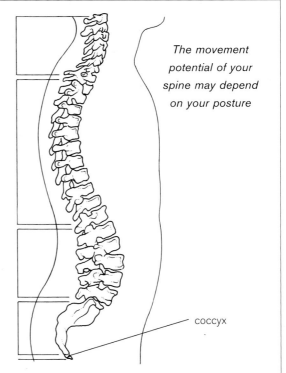

The cervical spine: the most mobile of all the spinal areas permitting all movements.

The thoracic spine: this is the least mobile of all the spinal areas due to the attachment of the ribs. There is little ability to bend forward or backward, but if you wish to twist or rotate, most of the action will take place here, especially in the section just above the hollow of your back.

The lumbar spine: here, rotation is very limited, but forward and backward bending (flexion and extension) occur mainly from this area.

The movement potential of your spine may depend on your posture

coccyx

sacrum

Action

1. Breathe in wide and full to prepare.
2. Breathe out, zipping up and hollowing, and slowly and carefully curl just the tailbone off the floor. You will lose the neutral pelvis position.
3. Breathe in, and breathe out, still zipping up and hollowing, as you lower and lengthen the spine back onto the floor.
4. Repeat, lifting a little more of the spine off the floor each time. As you lower, put each part of the spine down in sequence, bone by bone, aiming to put 'eight centimetres' between each vertebra. Replace them in this order: the back of the ribs, the waist, the small of the back and, finally, the tailbone.
5. You should complete five full curls, wheeling and lengthening the spine.

Watchpoints

- Take care that your back does not arch and that the tailbone stays tucked under like a whippet who has just been told off!
- Do not rush the first few curls. Really make the base of the spine move.
- There is a tendency sometimes, when there is a muscle imbalance in the torso, for one side to dominate. If you think of the spine 'landing' like a jet on a runway, it would often look as though you are landing in a high crosswind! Try to land down the central strip of the runway − no crosswinds!!!

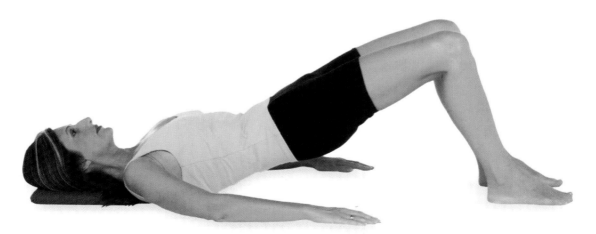

Full position

The Dart Stage Two ↻

Aim

To strengthen the back extensor muscles with trunk stability. To create awareness of the shoulder blades and to strengthen the muscles which stabilise them. To work the deep neck flexors.

Reminder of the Dart Stage One

Starting Position

* Lie on your front; you may place a flat pillow under your forehead to allow you to breathe.
* Your arms are down at your sides, your palms facing your body.
* Your neck is long.
* Your legs are together, in parallel, with your toes pointing.

Action

1. Breathe in to prepare and lengthen through the spine, tuck your chin in gently to hold that ripe peach.

2. Breathe out, zip up and hollow and pull your shoulder blades down into your back, lengthening your fingers away from you down towards your feet. The top of your head stays lengthening away from you.
3. Keep looking straight down at the floor. Do not tip your head back. Squeeze your inner thighs together but keep your feet on the floor.
4. Breathe in and feel the length of the body from the tips of your toes to the top of your head.
5. Breathe out, still zipping, and release.

The Dart Stage Two

When you have discovered the wonderful muscles that engage the shoulder blades down into the back, you may add lifting the upper body gently from the floor.

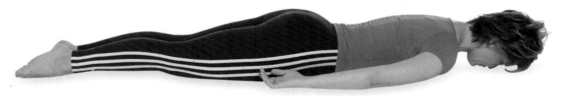

Start position

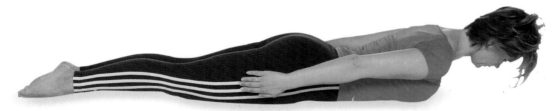

Stage Two

Action

1. Breathe in to prepare and lengthen through the spine, tucking your chin in gently.
2. Breathe out, zip up and hollow and pull your shoulder blades down into your back, lengthening your fingers away from you down towards your feet. The top of your head stays lengthening away from you.
3. Using the mid-back muscles, slowly raise the upper body from the floor. Keep looking straight down. Do not tip your head back. Squeeze your inner thighs together, but keep the feet on the floor.
4. Breathe in and feel the length of the body from the tips of your toes to the top of your head.
5. Breathe out, still zipped, and slowly lower.

Watchpoints

- Keep hollowing the lower abdominals.
- Do not strain the neck, it should feel released as your shoulders engage down into your back. Think of a swan's neck growing out between its wings.
- Please remember to keep your feet on the floor.
- Please stop if you feel at all uncomfortable in the low back. This exercise can also be done with the feet hip-width apart and the thigh and buttock muscles relaxed.

Rest Position

Aim

To lengthen and stretch out your sacral lumbar, middle and upper spine. To stretch your inner thighs. To make maximum use of the lungs, taking the breath into the back.

Please note: avoid the Rest Position if you have knee problems as you may compress the joint. You may like to place a cushion behind your knees to reduce this compression.

Action

Usually this exercise follows one in which you have been lying prone (on your front).

1. Come up onto all fours, bring your feet together, your knees stay apart. Slowly move back towards your buttocks. Do not raise your head or hands and come back to sit on your feet – not between them – with the back rounded.
2. Rest and relax into this position, leave the arms extended to give you a maximum stretch. Feel the expansion of the back of your ribcage as you breathe into it deeply.
3. The further apart the knees are the more of a stretch you will feel in your inner thighs. With the knees apart further, you can really think of your chest sinking down into the floor. You may also have the knees together which will increase the stretch for the lumbar spine.
4. Take ten breaths in this position.

To Come Out of the Rest Position

As you breathe out, zip up and hollow and slowly unfurl. Think of dropping your tailbone down and bringing your pubic bone forward. Rebuild your spine vertebra by vertebra until you are upright.

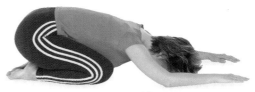

Rest Position

Pillow Squeeze ↻ 🏋

Aim

To isolate and work the pelvic floor in conjunction with the deep abdominals, engaging the deep stabilisers. To strengthen the inner thighs. To learn the correct position of the pelvis. To open the low back.

Equipment

Something to squeeze – a thick cushion, large towel or something of similar size. You may have to hunt around the gym or take your own cushion!

Starting Position

- Lie on your back. You may use a firm, flat cushion under your head if you wish. Have your feet together, flat on the floor.
- Place a cushion between your knees.
- Check that your pelvis is in neutral.

Action

1. Breathe in wide and full to prepare.
2. Breathe out and zip up and hollow.
3. Squeeze the cushion between your knees. Keep the pelvis in neutral, the tailbone down on the floor, lengthening away. Try not to grip around the hips.
4. Continue to breathe normally, squeezing and working the pelvic floor and deep abdominals, for a count of up to ten. Then release.
5. Repeat five times.

Watchpoints

- Do not hold your breath, keep breathing.
- Keep your neck released and your jaw soft. You do not need to use your neck to work the pelvic floor!
- The most common mistake made doing this exercise is to lift the tailbone and tuck the pelvis. Think of keeping the length in the front of the pelvis, do not curl or shorten it. Another good way to check if you are tilting is to place your hands under your waist. Try doing the exercise wrongly just once to feel the difference: you'll need to tuck the pelvis and feel the pressure on your hand – you are pushing into the spine. Now try to do the exercise with no pressure on the hand – you have stayed in neutral.

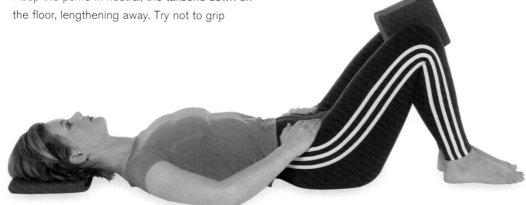

Pillow Squeeze

Gym Workouts

Repeating the same workout each time you visit the gym may not only lead to boredom but also to muscle imbalance. We need to challenge and stimulate ourselves constantly both mentally and physically. With this in mind we have given you seven gym workouts to choose from. They vary in length and give you the option of including an aerobic workout or not. If time, focus and energy are a problem we suggest you keep your aerobic and strength workouts separate.

We do not intend you to do one workout each day, it would be better to spread the workouts over a three- to four-week period. You should have two to three days' rest per week. Try not to repeat the same workout in succession and never workout when your muscles are tired or aching.

Remember the Six Golden Rules and the advice given on pages 21–41.

- Allow forty-eight to seventy-two hours between each weights or machine-based workout.
- Perform aerobic exercise three times a week, with a day or two in between. We give you an aerobic option for each workout so you will have to decide whether you wish to include this or not. Monitor your performance and recovery to what suits you.
- Perform two sets of each 'machine base' exercise to begin with. As you become stronger you may increase this to three sets.
- Perform eight repetitions on each set initially. When you can perform the exercise correctly and efficiently and remembering our key principles steadily increase your repetitions until you can reach twelve.
- Once you feel you can perform twelve repetitions comfortably then you can increase the resistance. Use the guide that the last two to three repetitions will be challenging without forcing you to perform poor and unsafe technique.
- Mentally absorb yourself fully into the exercise you are performing. Do not let your mind drift.
- If you wish, you may stretch or do non-weight-bearing Pilates exercises even in non-training days to keep the body supple.
- After a period of time you may hit a point of stagnation or tiredness. At this point it can be a good idea to take a week's break (no longer) from training. On your return you should feel refreshed and ready to re-start your programme. If stagnation continues after a break you may need to increase your intensity or apply some interesting changes to your routine.

- We recommend you use the 'Daily Workout Diary' (see example), or one similar, to record and monitor your progress.

PILATES GYM DAILY WORKOUT DIARY

WARM UP EXERCISES:				
AEROBIC OPTION: MACHINE TIME LEVEL OTHER				
EXERCISE	STRETCH	WEIGHT	REPS	SETS
PILATES EXERCISES:				

Workout One

Warm-up

Roll Downs	p. 46	
The Corkscrew	p. 49	
Waist Twists	p. 51	
Shoulder Circles	p. 48	
Neck Crescents	p. 50	
Five minutes on the rowing machine	p. 62	

Aerobic Option – *Pre-aerobic Stretches*

Standing Quadriceps Stretch	p. 54	
Lying Hamstring Stretch	p. 58	
Standing Calf Stretch	p. 60	
Standing Adductor Stretch	p. 61	
Up to twenty minutes on the bike. Use a heart-rate monitor if possible.	p. 64	
Cool down for three to five minutes to get your breath before moving onto the weights section.		
Side-lying Quadriceps Stretch	p. 56	

Machine Bases and Stretches

The Leg Press – two to three sets, eight to twelve repetitions	p. 72	
Standing Quadriceps Stretch	p. 54	
Hamstring Curls – two to three sets, eight to twelve repetitions	p. 74	
Lying Hamstring Stretch	p. 58	
Lat Pull Downs – two to three sets, eight to twelve repetitions	p. 76	
Lat Stretch	p. 78	
Chest Press two to three sets, eight to twelve repetitions	p. 82	
Pec Stretch: Through the Doorway	p. 87	
Shoulder Press – two to three sets, five repetitions	p. 88	
Shoulder Stretch	p. 90	
Triceps Push Downs – two to three sets, eight to twelve repetitions	p. 91	
Triceps Stretch	p. 93	
Seated Biceps Curls two to three sets, eight to twelve repetitions	p. 94	
Reverse Palm Stretch	p. 96	

Abductor Lifts	p. 151	
Adductor Lifts	p. 152	
Knee Stirs	p. 126	
Spine Curls	p. 106	
Side Rolls	p. 104	
Lying Hamstring Stretch	p. 58	

Adductor Stretch	p. 155	
Curl Ups with Leg Extension	p. 135	
Oblique Curl Ups	p. 99	
Diamond Press	p. 136	
Rest Position	p. 109	

Workout Two

Warm-up

Roll Downs	p. 46	
Waist Twists	p. 51	
The Corkscrew	p. 49	
Shoulder Circles	p. 48	
Neck Crescents	p. 50	
Five minutes on stationary bike	p. 64	

Aerobic Option – *Pre-aerobic Stretches*

Standing Quadriceps Stretch	p. 54	
Lying Hamstring Stretch	p. 58	
Standing Calf Stretch	p. 60	
Standing Adductor Stretch	p. 61	
Up to twenty minutes on the bike. Use a heart-rate monitor if possible.	p. 64	
Cool down for five minutes, by gradually slowing the pace to lower the heart rate.		
Side-lying Quadriceps Stretch	p. 56	

Main Workout

Side Rolls	p. 104	
Knee Stirs	p. 126	
Curl Ups	p. 98	
Oblique Curl Ups	p. 99	
Hip Flexor Stretch	p. 105	

Lying Hamstring Stretch (flex foot to introduce calf stretch)	p. 58	
Adductor Stretch	p. 155	
The Dart Stage Two	p. 108	
Rest Position	p. 109	
Pillow Squeeze	p. 110	

Workout Three

Warm-up

Roll Downs	p. 46	
Waist Twists	p. 51	
The Corkscrew	p. 49	
Shoulder Circles	p. 48	
Neck Crescents	p. 50	
Five minutes on cross trainer	p. 68	

Aerobic Option – *Pre-aerobic Stretches*

Standing Quadriceps Stretch	p. 54	
Lying Hamstring Stretch	p. 58	
Standing Calf Stretch	p. 60	
Standing Adductor Stretch	p. 61	
Up to twenty minutes on the treadmill. Use a heart-rate monitor if possible	p. 66	
Cool down by gradually reducing the pace for five minutes.		
Side-lying Quadriceps Stretch	p. 56	
Pliés – two to three sets, eight to twelve repetitions	p. 132	

Main Workout

Hamstring Scrunches (non machine) – two to three sets, eight to twelve repetitions	p. 154	
Lying Hamstring Stretch	p. 58	
Machine Rows – two to three sets, eight to twelve repetitions	p. 79	
Long Stretch	p. 81	
Push-ups (non-machine) – two to three sets, eight to twelve repetitions	p. 138, 139, 140	
Pec Stretch: Through the Doorway	p. 87	
Shoulder Press – two to three sets, five repetitions	p. 88	
Shoulder Stretch	p. 90	
Reverse Dips (non-machine) – two to three sets, eight to twelve repetitions	p. 134	
Triceps Stretch	p. 93	

Seated Biceps Curls (non-machine) – two to three sets, eight to twelve repetitions.	p. 94	
Reverse Palm Stretch.	p. 96	
Abductor Lifts	p. 150	
Adductor Lifts	p. 152	
Side Rolls	p. 104	
Spine Curls	p. 106	
Lying Hamstring Stretch	p. 58	
Side Reach and Side Stretch	p. 156	
Adductor Stretch	p. 155	
Single Leg Stretch	p. 100	
Oblique Curl Ups	p. 99	
Diamond Press	p. 136	
Rest Position	p. 109	

Workout Four

Warm-up

Shoulder Circles	p. 48	
Waist Twists	p. 51	
The Corkscrew	p. 49	
Neck Crescents	p. 50	
Five minutes on the treadmill	p. 66	

Aerobic Option – *Pre-aerobic Stretches*

Standing Quadriceps Stretch	p. 54	
Lying Hamstring Stretch	p. 58	
Standing Calf Stretch	p. 60	
Standing Adductor Stretch	p. 61	
Twenty-minute power walk on treadmill (jog or run if you are already aerobically fit). Use a heart-rate monitor if possible	p. 66	
Cool down by reducing the pace for five minutes. Walk on treadmill to lower heart rate.		
Side-lying Quadriceps Stretch	p. 56	

Main Workout

Pelvic Stability Check	p. 34	
Spine Curls	p. 106	
Hip Flexor Stretch	p. 105	
Windows	p. 129	
Side Rolls	p. 104	
Curl Ups with Leg Extension	p. 135	
Oblique Single Leg Stretch	p. 102	
The Dart Stage Two	p. 108	
Rest Position	p. 109	
Roll Downs	p. 46	

Workout Five

Warm-up

Roll Downs	p.46	
The Corkscrew	p.49	
Shoulder Circles	p.48	
Neck Crescents	p.50	
Five minutes on rowing machine (use a heartrate monitor if possible)	p.62	

Aerobic Option – *Pre-aerobic Stretches*

Standing Quadriceps Stretch	p. 54	
Lying Hamstring Stretch	p. 58	
Standing Calf Stretch	p. 60	
Standing Adductor Stretch	p. 61	
Up to twenty minutes on the cross-training machine. Use a heart-rate monitor if possible	p. 68	
Side-lying Quadriceps Stretch	p. 56	

Machine Bases

Leg Press – two to three sets, eight to twelve repetitions.	p. 72	
Standing Quadriceps Stretch	p. 54	
Hamstring Scrunch (non machine) – two to three sets, eight to twelve repetitions.	p. 154	
Lat Pull Downs – two to three sets, eight to twelve repetitions	p. 76	
Lat Stretch	p. 78	
Shoulder Press – two to three sets, five repetitions	p. 88	
Shoulder Stretch	p. 90	
Pec Deck – two to three sets, eight to twelve repetitions	p. 85	
Pec Deck Stretch	p. 84	
Seated Biceps Curls – two to three sets, eight to twelve repetitions	p. 94	
Reverse Palm Stretch	p.96	
Abductor Lifts	p.150	
Adductor Lifts	p.152	
Side Rolls	p.104	

Spine Curls	p. 106	
Lying Hamstring Stretch	p. 58	
Arm Openings	p. 158	
Knee Stirs	p. 126	

Adductor Stretch	p. 155	
Diamond Press	p. 136	
Rest Position	p. 109	

Workout Six

Warm-up

Shoulder Circles	p. 48	
Waist Twists	p. 51	
Neck Crescents	p. 50	
Walking on the Spot	p. 52	
Five minutes on the treadmill	p. 66	

Aerobic Option – *Pre-aerobic Stretches*

Standing Quadriceps Stretch	p. 54	
Lying Hamstring Stretch	p. 58	
Standing Calf Stretch	p. 60	
Standing Adductor Stretch	p. 61	
Up to twenty minutes on the cross-training machine. Use a heart-rate monitor if possible	p.68	
Side-lying Quadriceps Stretch	p.56	

Main Workout

Lying Hamstring Stretch	p. 58	
Spine Curls	p. 106	
Hip Flexor Stretch	p. 105	
Side Rolls	p. 104	
The Pelvic Bridge	p. 128	

Push-ups (non-machine) – two to three sets, eight to twelve repetitions	p. 138, 139, 140	
The Dart	p. 38	
Rest Position	p. 109	
Roll Downs	p. 46	
Pillow Squeeze	p. 110	

Workout Seven

Warm-up

Roll Downs	p. 46	
The Corkscrew	p. 49	
Shoulder Circles	p. 48	
Neck Crescents	p. 50	
Five minutes on the rowing machine to warm-up.	p. 62	

Aerobic Option – *Pre-aerobic Stretches*

Long Stretch (see Machine Rows)	p. 81	
Standing Quadriceps Stretch	p. 54	
Lying Hamstring Stretch	p. 58	
Standing Calf Stretch	p. 60	
Standing Adductor Stretch	p. 61	
Up to twenty minutes on the rowing machine – work steadily and progressively as you may fatigue quickly to begin with. Use a heart-rate monitor if possible. Five minutes on treadmill to cool down and lower heart rate.		
Side-lying Quadriceps Stretch	p. 56	

Main Workout

Spine Curls	p. 106	
Hip Flexor Stretch	p. 105	
Side Rolls	p. 104	
Curl Ups with Leg Extension	p. 135	
Oblique Curl Ups	p. 99	

The Dart Stage Two	p. 108	
Diamond Press	p. 136	
Rest Position	p. 109	
Side Reach and Side Stretch	p.156	
Pillow Squeeze see	p. 110	

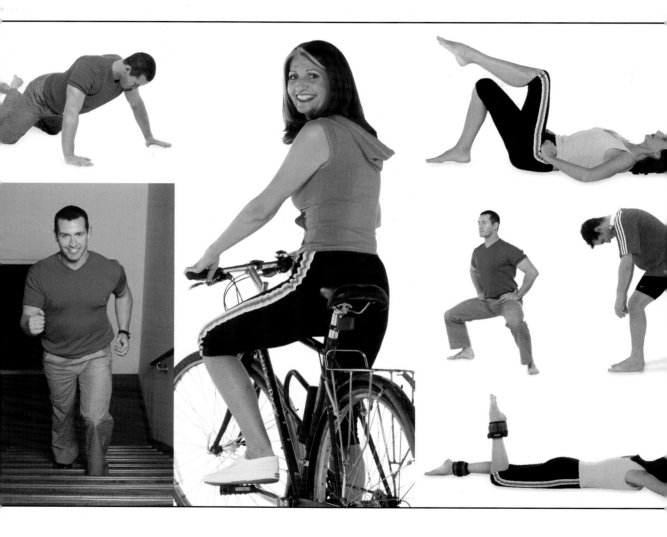

Home Gym

In this section, we have put together a series of exercises for when you can't get to the gym. As with the gym workout, variety is the key to a balanced programme. After a short warm-up, we suggest you do five minutes of aerobic activity before embarking on the main workout, which includes both stretching and strengthening work as well as exercises that promote joint mobility and good movement patterns. You may also wish to include the abdominal exercises on page 98–102.

We recommend that three times a week you should increase aerobic activity to twenty minutes.

At the end of this chapter, you will find seven home workouts to try.

Warm-up

Remove your shoes for the mat excercise in this home programme.

Aerobic Warm-up

Shoes back on as you spend five minutes on an aerobic activity to raise your heart rate and body temperature gently. As soon as your heart rate has recovered you may then move on to the main home workout. Remove your shoes again.

Main Workout

This includes exercises to establish sound movement patterns and to increase flexibility and joint mobility.

Weights and Stretches

These exercises are designed to increase strength in the arms and legs.

Adding Aerobic Training

At least three times a week, aim to spend twenty minutes on aerobic training which you can do either before or after your main workout or separately if you wish. If possible perform aerobic exercise on separate days.

You need to warm-up before you start by doing the following stretches:

Standing Quadriceps Stretch see page 54
Lying Hamstring Stretch see page 58
Standing Calf Stretch see page 60
Standing Adductor Stretch see page 61

These stretches may also be done after the aerobic session. You may also like to add the Side-lying Quadriceps Stretch see page 56.

Choose from the following for your aerobic session:

Running
Cycling
Skipping
Rebounder
Power walking/hiking
Stationary bike
Home rower
Aerobics video

Wind-down

These exercises should be done at the end of each workout to rebalance the body.

Warm-up

Your warm-up consists of six exercises, some of which will be familiar from the Gym Workout section, followed by five minutes of gentle aerobic work to raise your body temperature and heart rate. Four of the exercises have been described earlier:

> Spine Curls see page 106
> Side Rolls see page 104
> Hip Flexor Stretch see page 105
> Neck Rolls/Chin Tucks see page 27

Shoulder Drops

Aim
To release tension in the upper body, gently mobilising the shoulders.

Starting Position
- Lie in the Relaxation Position.

Action
1. Raise both arms towards the ceiling directly above your shoulders, palms facing each other.
2. Reach for the ceiling with one arm, stretch through the fingertips. The shoulder blade comes off the floor. Then drop the arm back down onto the floor.
3. Repeat ten times with each arm. Feel your upper back widening and the tension in your shoulders releasing down into the floor.

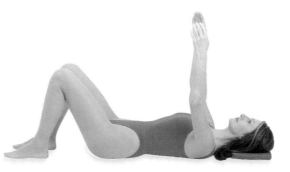

Shoulder Drops

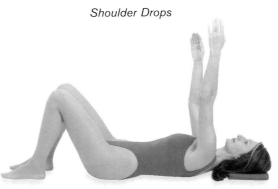

Knee Stirs 🚲 ↻

Aim

To release the muscles around the hip. To promote hip mobility and pelvic stability.

Starting Position

- Lie in the Relaxation Position – place your hands on your pelvis to check it stays still.
- You may either wrap a scarf around one thigh, holding it from underneath so that the shoulders stay down and relaxed, or do the exercise without a scarf as shown below.
- Fold the knee up, so that it is directly above the hip.

Action

1. Keeping the pelvis neutral and stable – do not allow it to rock from side to side – gently and slowly circle the bent leg around.
2. Breathe normally as you do so, zipping up and hollowing throughout.
3. Think of releasing the thigh bone from the hip socket. If you are using the scarf allow the scarf (and your hands) to help move the leg.
4. Circle five times clockwise, five anti-clockwise with each leg.

Watchpoints

- Check that holding the scarf hasn't created tension in the upper body. If it has, try the exercise without the scarf, but still maintaining the sense of openness in the hip.
- Keep checking that your pelvis is in neutral, tailbone down and lengthening away.
- Don't take the leg too wide to begin with – initially the circle should be the size of a grapefruit. You may take it wider as you become more confident.

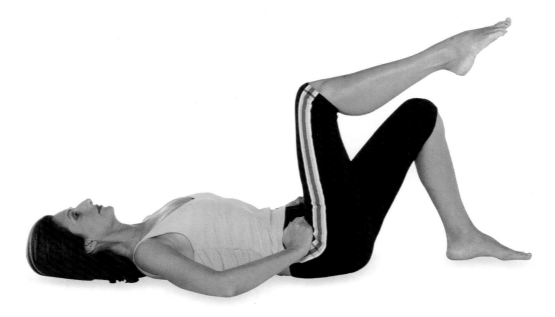

Main Workout

There are eleven exercises in this section.

Pelvic Stability Check ↻

Aim
To check the stability of your pelvis.

Starting Position
- Lie in the Relaxation Position. Your pelvis is in neutral, it should remain in neutral throughout the exercise. Place your hands on your lower abdomen, to check that your muscles stay hollow without bulging.

Action
1. Breathe in wide and full to prepare.
2. Breathe out, zip up and hollow and fold one knee towards your chest, dropping the thigh bone down into the hip socket. Breathe in and check you are still in neutral.
3. Breathe out, still zipped, and extend the leg at about an angle of 45° into the air, keeping your lower abdominals hollowed and your pelvis still.
4. Breathe in as the leg bends up again and breathe out as you return the leg to the floor.
5. Repeat five times with each leg.

Watchpoints
- Maintain neutral pelvis throughout.
- Use your hands to check that your lower abdominals stay hollow.
- Keep both sides of your waist long.

Start position

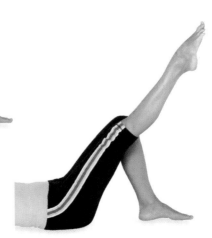

Full position

The Pelvic Bridge ↻

Aim

To learn pelvic stability and to strengthen the buttocks.

This isn't as easy as it looks and requires good abdominals and back muscles. If you find yourself wobbling, you may not be ready yet, so practise the exercises on page 98–102 for a while longer.

Starting Position

- Lie in the Relaxation Position, your feet together, about twenty centimetres from your buttocks.
- Leave your arms by your sides, palms down.

Action

1. Breathe in wide and full to prepare.
2. Breathe out, zipping up and hollowing and slowly lift your lower body from the floor, keeping your pelvis in neutral. (Unlike for Spine Curls your body rises like a plane taking off.)
3. Breathe normally as you check that your spine is now in a neutral position and bring your hands to rest on your pelvis.
4. On your next out-breath, still zipping and hollowing, straighten one leg, keeping the knees together so that the leg extends in a straight line. Keep your pelvis completely still, do not allow it to dip. Think of keeping both sides of your waist long.

5. Breathe in and return the foot to the floor.
6. Work up to repeating the exercise five times with each leg before lowering your body back down onto the floor.

Watchpoints

- There is sometimes a tendency, when there is a muscle imbalance in the torso, for one side to dominate. As you lift and lower the spine, think of a jet taking off and landing right down the central strip of the runway. No high crosswind!
- Check constantly that, as you extend your leg, your pelvis stays in neutral north, south, east and west.
- Use your hands to check for movement in the pelvis. They will also automatically help to keep you a little more stable.

Moving On

To make this exercise harder, take your hands away from your pelvis and fold them easily across your chest. This reduces your base of support which means that you have to work harder to stabilise.

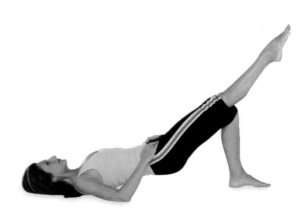

Start position   *Full position*

Windows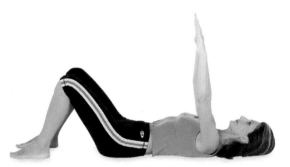

Aim

To promote flexibility and mobility around the shoulder joint.

Please take advice if you have a shoulder injury.

Stage one

Starting Position

- Lie in the Relaxation Position.
- Raise your arms directly above your shoulders, palms facing away from you, your shoulder blades remain down into your back, your upper body relaxed and open.

Action

1. Breathe in wide and full to prepare.
2. Breathe out, zip up and hollow. Stay zipped now and bring your elbows down towards the floor, keeping your arms bent. Your upper arms are now in a line with the shoulders to each side.

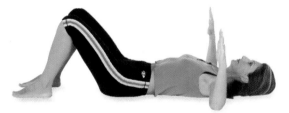

Stage two

3. Breathe in and very slowly rotate your arms backwards. The backs of your hands will come down towards the floor. Under no circumstances force the arms back, stop where they are comfortable. Feel your shoulder blades connecting down into your back as you make this movement.
4. Breathe out as you straighten the arms slowly, keeping them wide and keeping the shoulder blades down in your back.
5. Breathe in as you raise the arms back to the Starting Position.
6. Repeat eight times.

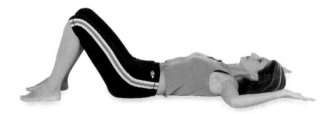

Stage three

Watchpoints

- Make your movements smooth, controlled, without strain.
- Shoulder blades down at all times.
- Keep your ribcage and your breastbone soft.

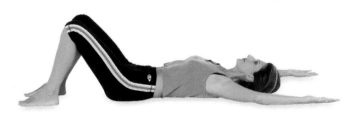

Stage four

Roll Downs Against a Wall ↻ 🚴 🤸

Aim

To release tension in the spine, the shoulders and the upper body. To mobilise the spine, creating flexibility and strength and achieving segmental control. To teach correct use of stabilising abdominals when bending.

Please take advice if you have a back problem (see below), especially if it is disc-related.

This fabulous exercise can be used during your warm-up or your wind-down with equal effect. It combines stabilising work with the wonderful wheeling motion of the spine.

As you roll back up think of rebuilding the spinal column, stacking each vertebra on top of each other to lengthen out the spine.

Starting Position

*   Stand about forty-five centimetres from a wall – the distance really depends on your height, but you should feel comfortable.
*   Your knees are bent so that from the side you look as if you are sitting on a bar stool!
*   Have your feet hip-width apart and in parallel, your weight evenly balanced on both feet. Check that you are not rolling your feet in or out.
*   Find your neutral pelvis position, but keep the tailbone lengthening down.

Action

1. Breathe in to prepare and lengthen up through the spine, release the head and neck.
2. Breathe out, zip up and hollow, drop your chin onto your chest and allow the weight of your head to make you roll slowly forward, head released, arms hanging, centre strong, knees soft . If you have a back problem, you may like

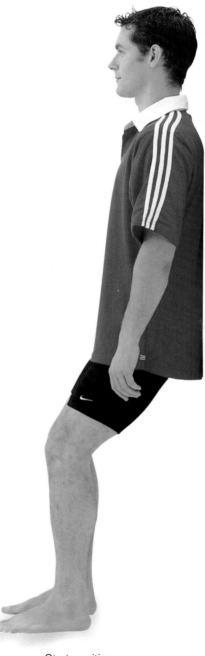

Start position

to begin by sliding your hands down your thighs.

3. Breathe in as you hang, really letting your head and arms hang.

4. Breathe out and firmly zip up and hollow as you drop your tailbone down, directing your pubic bone forward. Rotate your pelvis backwards as you come up the wall slowly, rolling through the spine bone by bone.

5. Repeat six times.

Watchpoints

• You may like to take an extra breath during the exercise. This is fine, but please try to breathe out as you move the spine.

• Make sure that you go down centrally and do not sway over to one side. When you are down, check where your hands are in relation to your feet.

• Do not roll the feet in or out. Keep the weight evenly balanced and try not to lean forward onto the front of your feet or back onto the heels.

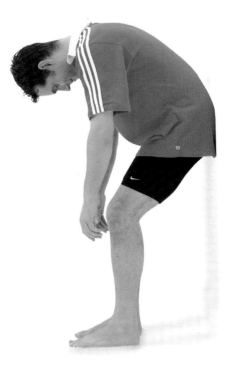

Stage one

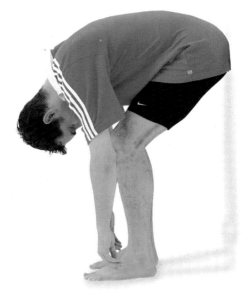

Stage two

Pliés ♉

Aim

To strengthen and shape the quadriceps, gluteus maximus and adductor muscles.

Starting Position

- Ideally you should stand in front of a mirror to monitor your technique.
- Your feet should be placed slightly wider than shoulder-width apart. The toes should be pointing outward at a 45° angle.
- Place your hands on your hips.

Action

1. Breathe in wide and full to prepare and lengthen through the spine.
2. Breathe out, zip up and hollow and, maintaining pelvic and spinal neutral, bend your knees directly over the centre of your feet. Bend as far as you are comfortable, but not beyond a 90° angle.
3. Breathe in wide and full and hold the plié.

4. Breathe out as you push up through the thighs, really using the inner thighs but keeping them long and straightening up at end of the movement.

Watchpoints

- Keep all your movements smooth and controlled.
- Keep the shoulder blades down into the back and the neck long.
- Keep zipping up and hollowing throughout, pelvis neutral, spine lengthened and the tail-bone lengthening away. It is easy to lose these points during this exercise.
- Avoid locking the knees as you return to the Starting Position.
- Avoid tipping the upper body forward on the downward movement.

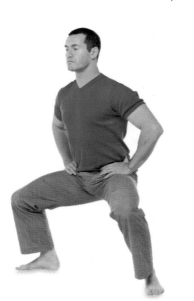

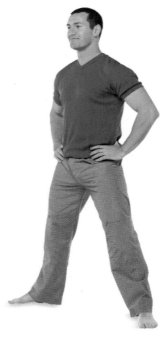

Back Scrub 🕴 🚲

Aim

To promote shoulder mobility and also strength and flexibility in the upper arms.

Starting Position

- Stand correctly, holding a long rolled towel or scarf in your right hand.

Action

1. Breathe in wide and full to prepare.
2. As you breathe out, zip up and hollow (stay zipped now), take your right hand over and behind your head, your left hand under and behind your back so that you are able to grasp the bottom of the towel.
3. Breathe normally now, as you slide the towel up and down as if scrubbing your back.
4. Repeat ten times, making sure that you do not arch your back or twist your neck.
5. Gently release the towel from underneath and repeat on the other side.

Watchpoints

- Try to keep your shoulder blades down into your back throughout the action.
- Keep your neck in the centre, long and released.
- Keep checking that you are standing well – imagine a small weight attached to your tail-bone to help keep good neutral alignment.
- Your chest will open but try not to allow your ribs to flare.

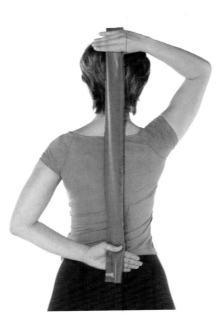

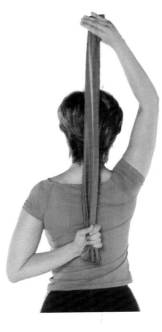

Reverse Dips

Aim

To strengthen and shape the triceps.

Starting Position

- Ideally, position yourself side-on to a mirror so that you can check your alignment.
- Sit on the end of a workout bench or chair. Place your hands on the ends of the bench or chair, fingers facing forward. Lift your bottom off the end of the bench and walk your feet forward until your knees are in line with your ankles.

Action

1. Breathe in wide and full to prepare and lengthen up through the spine.
2. Breathe out, zip up and hollow. Stay zipped now, keeping your pelvis in neutral and bend the elbows under control to a 90 ° angle.
3. Breathe in and breathe out as you return to the Starting Position.
5. Repeat up to ten times.

Watchpoints

- Keep all your movements smooth and controlled.
- Keep the shoulder blades down into the back. Your neck should be long and the back of your head in line with your spine.
- Keep zipping up and hollowing throughout, the pelvis neutral, spine lengthened and the tail-bone lengthened away.
- Avoid locking the elbow joints on the upward movement.
- Do not allow the body to move too far away from the bench or chair. This puts stress on the shoulder joints and shortens the neck.

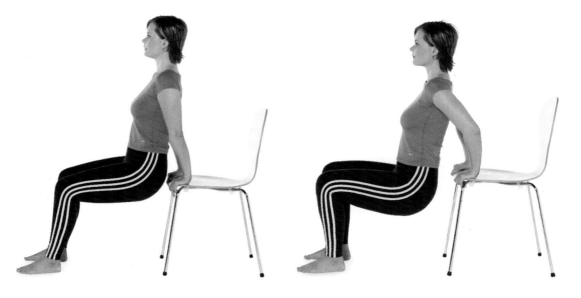

Start position   *Full position*

Curl Ups with Leg Extension ↻

The additional challenge of extending your leg while curling up really helps to target the lower abdominals. Follow the directions very carefully to see dramatic results.

Please note: avoid this exercise if you have neck problems.

Aim

To strengthen the abdominals with the added challenge of leg extension.

Starting Position

- Lie on your back with your knees bent, feet together and in parallel. You may like a flat pillow under your head.
- Gently release your neck by rolling the head slowly from side to side.
- Place your hands behind your head, elbows open (you should still be able to see them).
- Make sure that your pelvis is in its neutral position, neither tucked nor arched.

Action

1. Breathe in wide and full to prepare. Gently tuck your chin in as if holding, but not squashing, a large ripe peach.
2. Breathe out, zip up and hollow. Without tilting the pelvis, soften your breastbone and curl up breaking from the breastbone. As you do so, slowly extend your right leg, keeping the right knee in line with your left knee and your thighs also in a line. Your stomach must not pop up. Keep the length and width in the front of the pelvis and the tailbone down on the floor lengthening away. Do not tuck the pelvis or pull on the neck!
3. Breathe in, still zipped up and slowly curl back down, bending the knee at the same time.
4. Repeat ten times with each leg changing over hands halfway through.

Watchpoints

- Try not to grip around the hips.
- Stay in neutral, tailbone down on the floor and lengthening away. A useful image is that there is a strip of sticky tape along the front of the body that should not wrinkle!

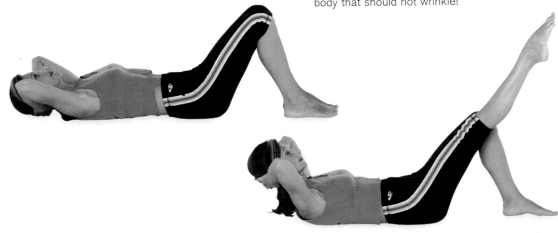

Diamond Press C 🚴 🤸

Aim

To develop awareness of the shoulder blades moving on the ribcage. To work the muscles that stabilise the shoulder blades, especially lower trapezius. To work the deep neck flexors. To encourage lengthening, while extending the back.

A subtle exercise which has dramatic results. It really does help to reverse the effects of being 'hunched over' all day. You can feel the tension in your neck release as the stabilising muscles work.

Starting Position

- Lie on your front with your feet hip-width apart and parallel.
- Create a diamond shape with your arms by placing your fingertips together just above your forehead. Your elbows are open, your shoulder blades relaxed.

Action

1. Breathe in and lengthen through the spine.
2. Breathe out, zip up and hollow and pull the shoulder blades down into the back of your waist. Gently tuck your chin in and lift your head three or four centimetres off the floor. Stay looking down at the floor; the back of the neck is long. Imagine a cord pulling you from the top of your head. Really make the connection down into the small of your back – you have to push a little on the elbows, but think of them connecting with your waist as well.
3. Breathe in and hold the position. Keep the lower abdominals hollowed but the ribs stay on the floor.
4. Breathe out, still zipped, and slowly lower back down. Keep lengthening through the spine.
5. Repeat five times.

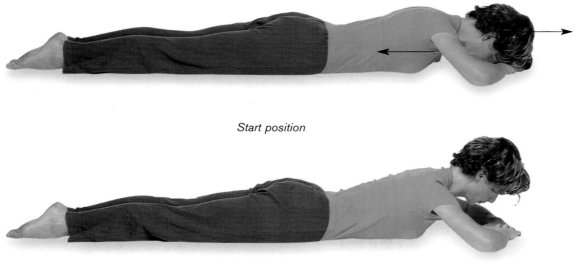

Start position

Full position

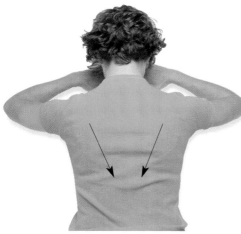

Full position – from above

Watchpoints

- Keep the lower abdominals drawing back to the spine.
- Make sure that you keep looking down at the floor – if you lift your head back you will shorten the back of the neck.

After the Diamond Press come into the Rest Position see page 109.

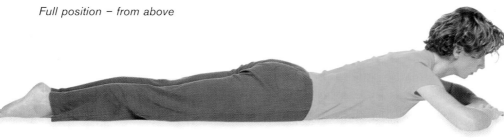

Incorrect position – do not throw your head back

Push-ups

Aim

To strengthen and shape the pectoral, deltoid and triceps muscles and the wrists.

We are going to give you three levels for this exercise. The first is very gentle but teaches you technique as well as gradually improving your upper-body and wrist strength. Once this becomes easy, you can progress to the Intermediate version and then, finally, the full Advanced Push-up.

Push-ups Against a Wall (Beginner's Level)

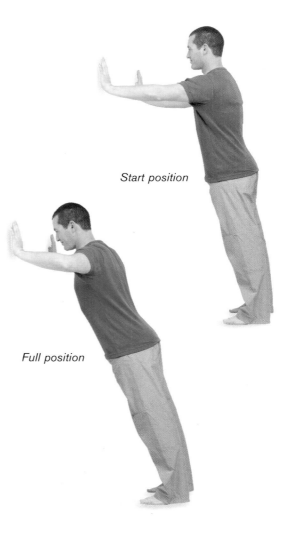

Start position

Full position

Starting Position

- Stand facing a wall, about forty-five centimetres away (the further away you are the harder the exercise).
- Place your palms on the wall at about shoulder height but slightly wider than your shoulders.
- Have your feet hip-width apart and parallel.

Action

1. Breathe in to prepare.
2. Breathe out, zip up and hollow (stay zipped now) and slowly lower your body towards the wall, allowing your elbows to open, but keeping your shoulder blades down into your back.
3. Breathe in and push yourself away from the wall again.
4. Repeat up to ten times.

Watchpoints

- Keep your shoulder blades down in your back throughout the exercise – really try to feel the connection.
- Keep your neck long and released.
- Do not lock your elbows.

Push-ups (Intermediate Level)

Starting Position

- Come onto all fours, have your hands at shoulder level but slightly wider than your shoulders. Fingers facing forward. Your knees should be further away from your hips (see photo), hip-width apart, with your ankles crossed.
- Look straight down at the floor to keep the back of your neck long.
- Throughout the exercise your pelvis and spine remain in neutral.

Action

1. Breathe in wide and full to prepare.
2. Breathe out, zip up and hollow (stay zipped now) and slowly lower your upper body down towards the floor, keeping a long and neutral spine. You pivot on your knees.
3. Breathe in as you slowly straighten your arms.
4. Work up to ten repetitions.

Watchpoints

- Keep your shoulder blades down in your back throughout the exercise, really try to feel the connection.
- Keep your neck long and released.
- Do not lock your elbows.

Moving On

To make the exercise more challenging, move your knees further back, until you have the strength to do the full push-up.

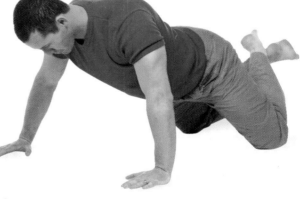

Start position

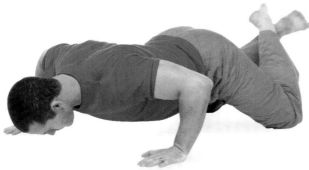

Full position

Push-ups (Advanced Level)

This exercise requires a great deal of upper-body strength and core stability to be performed safely and effectively.

Starting Position

- Place your hands just wider than shoulder-width apart – palms down and fingers facing forward.
- Raise your knees from the floor and come up onto the balls of your feet.

Action

1. Breathe in wide and full to prepare and lengthen through the spine.
2. Breathe out, zipping and hollowing. Stay zipped and maintaining pelvic and spinal neutral, bend the elbows in a controlled movement to a 90° angle. Your chest should finish just above the floor.
3. Breathe in.
4. Breathe out as you push up until the arms are straight.

Watchpoints

- Keep zipped up and hollowed throughout, pelvis neutral, spine lengthened and the tailbone lengthening away.
- Keep the shoulder blades down into the back and your chin tucked gently in. The back of your head should be in line with your spine.
- Ensure that you do not lock the elbow joints at the top part of the movement.

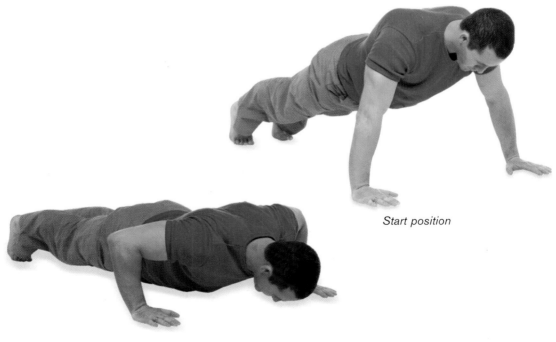

Start position

Full position

Weights and Stretches

This next set of exercises has been designed to replace the workout you would get if you were using gym equipment. They will help tone and strengthen your muscles. As with the exercises on machine bases, you do need to do some flexibility work after using weights. All of these exercises can be done without weights at all. In fact, we recommend that you attempt them first without weights to perfect your technique and slowly build your muscle strength.

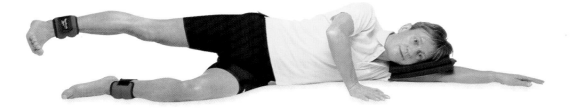

The following set of exercises has been designed to help tone and strengthen your muscles.

If You Don't Have Weights

Making your own weights is easy. Instead of hand-held weights you use cans of beans or bags of rice.

To make your own leg weights take an old, clean pair of thick tights. Cut the legs off. About fifteen centimetres from the toes tie a knot. Then weigh out between 0.5–1.5 kilograms of rice (uncooked) and pour into the tights. Tie another knot about twenty centimetres away from the first knot. Now you have a set of weights that you can tie onto your ankles. A word of caution, however – pick a pair of tights with no holes or all the rice trickles through! Fishnet tights are not recommended for this.

Normally we recommend that you use arm weights of up to two kilos each weight. However, if you wish to use heavier weights you may, but you must never strain and you must still be able to stabilise. If you find your movements becoming jerky, then the weight is too heavy. Each leg weight should be below one kilo.

Arm Weights

Backstroke Swimming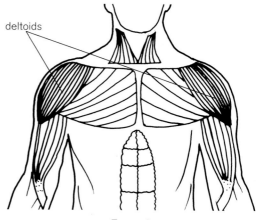

Aim

To learn correct shoulder movement, stabilising the shoulder blades. To open the shoulder blades. To combat round shoulders. To work the adductors and inner thighs.

A wonderful exercise to counter those hunched positions we all find ourselves in every day. Enjoy the sensation of opening out.

Equipment

Hand-weights of between 0.5 and 1 kilo. Do not use heavier weights for this exercise. Tennis ball or pillow.

deltoids

Front view

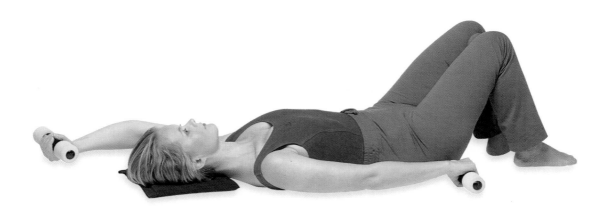

Full position

Starting Position

- Lie on a narrow bench, if possible.
- Lie in the Relaxation Position, but this time bring your feet together lined up perfectly, a tennis ball placed between the knees. Your feet are flat on the floor.
- Holding the hand weights, raise your arms to the ceiling, palms away from your face with your elbows slightly bent.
- Throughout the exercise, you will be zipping up and hollowing and squeezing the pillow or tennis ball gently.

Action

1. Breathe in wide and full to prepare.
2. Breathe out, zip up and hollow, as you take the right arm behind you to the floor and the left hand down to the side of your hip.
3. Breathe in as you bring the arms back up to the Starting Position.
4. Breathe out as you repeat the movement to the other side.
5. Keep squeezing the inner thighs and hollowing the lower abdominals.
6. Repeat ten times to each side.

Watchpoints

- Neutral pelvis please.
- As you take the arm behind you, keep it outside the line of the shoulder.
- If you are using a bench, keep the arm in line with the body and parallel to your side.
- Keep squeezing the inner thighs together, but don't lift the tailbone.
- Keep a sense of openness in the upper body and keep those shoulder blades engaged down into the back.

Flies

Aim

To open the upper body, teaching correct upper-body use. To tone the chest and upper-arm muscles. To work the inner thighs. To increase bone density.

Equipment

Arm weights – increase the weight as you become stronger. Tennis ball or pillow.

Starting Position

- Lie on your back, knees bent and together. Put the tennis ball between the knees. Feet flat.
- Extend the arms upwards, keeping the natural shape of the arm with the elbows slightly bent, as if you are hugging a large tree trunk.
- Throughout the exercise you will be zipping up and hollowing, squeezing the pillow or tennis ball gently, pelvis in neutral of course.

Action

1. Breathe in as you open the arms directly to the side down onto the floor, keeping their natural shape. The elbows stay slightly bent.
2. Breathe out as you bring the arms back above your chest in line with your breastbone.
3. Keep squeezing the inner thighs together and hollowing out the lower abdominals.
4. Repeat ten times.

Watchpoints

- Don't unfold the arms, i.e. don't hinge from the elbow – keep the natural curve.
- Take the arms directly to the side, rather than taking the weight behind you.
- Keep hollowing the abdominals – remember north to south, neutral spine.
- Keep squeezing those inner thighs, but don't lift the tailbone – keep it lengthening away.

Start position

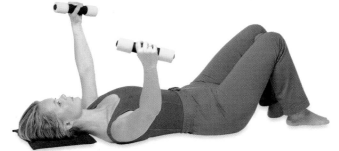

Full position

Biceps

Aim

To strengthen the bicep muscles, while stabilising the shoulder blades. To strengthen the muscles that pronate and supernate (rotate) your elbow.

Equipment

Hand-held weights of up to 2.5 kilos each weight.

Starting Position

*   Stand correctly, reminding yourself of all the directions on page 26.
*   Hold the weight in one hand, palm facing your thigh. Take your other hand across and lightly hold your arm just above the elbow.

Action

1. Breathe in wide and full to prepare, lengthening up through the spine.
2. Breathe normally now and, as you raise the arm, gently and slowly rotate your forearm inwards and outwards keeping the elbow quite still and close into your side. Your hand will finish close to your shoulder joint.
3. Breathe in as you return it to your side.
4. Repeat five times with each arm.

Watchpoints

*   Keep the elbow isolated and still.
*   Keep reminding yourself of the correct standing instructions, lengthening up through the spine.
*   Keep your shoulder blade down into your back, and your upper body open.
*   Try not to allow your wrist to go floppy.

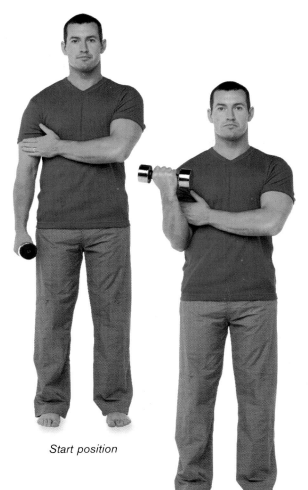

Start position

Full position

Triceps

Aim

To strengthen the triceps without compromising the neck. If using a cushion, to strengthen the inner thighs.

There are lots of ways to work the triceps. This one is great because there is no risk of over-using your neck muscles. You will need to take a firm grip on the weight.

Equipment

A weight. You may also need a cushion or tennis ball.

Starting Position

- Lie with your knees bent, pelvis in neutral. If you wish, you may place a small cushion or tennis ball between your knees and throughout the exercise you can squeeze the cushion to work the inner thighs (not shown below).
- Hold the weight firmly in your right hand and take the weight up and across so that it is above your left shoulder. The idea is for the upper part of the right arm to be straight and directly above your right shoulder.
- Gently support your right elbow with your left hand (see photo below).
- Take a moment to check that your shoulder blades are down into your back and that your upper body is relaxed and open.

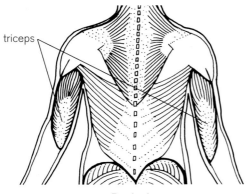

Back view

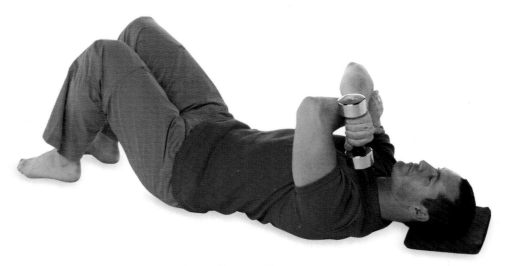

Start position

Action

1. Breathe in to prepare.
2. Breathe out, zip up and hollow and slowly straighten your arm, keeping the elbow quite still. Do not fully straighten the arm, stop just short.
3. Breathe in as you lower.
4. Repeat up to twenty times.

Watchpoints

- Keep that firm grip on the weight.
- Keep your neck released and your shoulder blades down into your back.
- If you are squeezing the cushion between your knees, be sure that you do not tilt the pelvis or grip around the hips – see Pillow Squeeze on page 110.

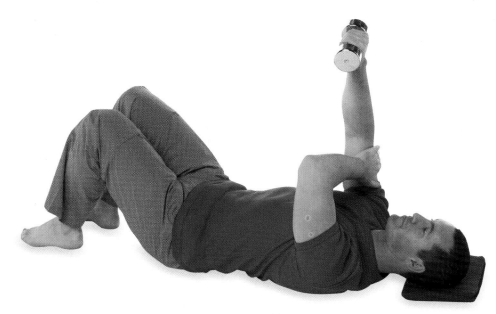

Full position

Upper-body Stretches

Wall Stretch One

Aim

To stretch between the shoulders and around the arms.

These exercises really do reach parts that others cannot reach. Follow the instructions carefully, take good note of the positions shown in the photographs, but you may have to adjust your own position fractionally to get at the tight areas. These are powerful stretches, so please treat them with respect.

Please consult your practitioner if you have a shoulder, hip or knee injury.

Starting Position

- Sit facing a wall, have your legs crossed comfortably. If you cannot cross your legs you can do this exercise standing but the stretch will be less. The further away from the wall you are the more of a stretch you will feel.
- Place your palms on the wall above you, wider than your shoulders, elbows open, shoulder blades down into your back.

Action

1. Breathe in to prepare.
2. Breathe out and zip up and hollow (stay zipped now).
3. Breathe normally as you lean into the wall. You should feel the stretch between your shoulder blades and possibly in your upper arms and around your hips.

4. Hold the stretch for about thirty seconds, before releasing.
5. Repeat five times.

Watchpoints

- Keep your neck long and released.
- Your upper back is slightly extended in this position, so keep all the stabilising muscles working.

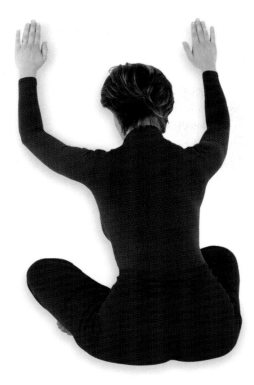

Wall Stretch Two 🏃

Aim

To stretch and open the upper body.

You must keep lengthening upwards in this exercise and not collapse.

Please consult your practitioner if you have a shoulder, hip or knee injury.

Starting Position

- Sit comfortably crossed-legged with your right side onto a wall. If you cannot cross your legs you can do this exercise standing but the stretch will be less.
- Place your hands on the wall, out to the sides, at shoulder height.

Action

1. Breathe in to prepare and lengthen up through the spine.
2. As you breathe out, zip up and hollow (stay zipped now) and slowly turn your upper body towards the wall, pushing a little on your right hand.
3. Breathe normally as you hold the stretch, which you should feel between the shoulder blade and the spine on your right side. Hold the stretch for about thirty seconds.
4. Repeat three times before turning around to stretch the other side.

Watchpoints

- Keep lengthening up out of your hips.
- The stretch should be felt but not be uncomfortable, it's a sort of delicious pain!
- Keep your shoulder blades down into your back and your neck released.

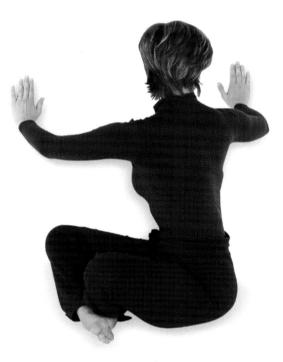

Leg Weights

Practise these exercises first without weights, until you are totally familiar with them and they cause you no discomfort. When you do move on to use the weights they should be placed on the ankles. It is easier to complete all the leg-weight exercises on one side and then turn over to do them on the other side.

Abductor Lifts

Aim

To strengthen the abductors (outer thigh) and the gluteals. It also tones the upper leg and controls cellulite.

This and Twenty Lifts will challenge your pelvic and lumbar stability so you must be stable before attempting them. Good preparation exercises are the pelvic stability exercises.

Equipment

Pillow. Leg weights. Piece of foam or small flat pillow (optional).

Starting Position

- Lie on your right side in a straight line, but maintaining your natural curves – this is crucial, so, if you like, you can lie up against a wall to check your alignment. Don't lean on the wall! Remember neutral please.
- Your right arm is stretched out, your head resting against the arm. You may place a pillow between your ear and your arm so that the head is at the right angle to the spine.
- Bend both legs in front of you at an angle of just under 90°. Use your left arm to support yourself in front.

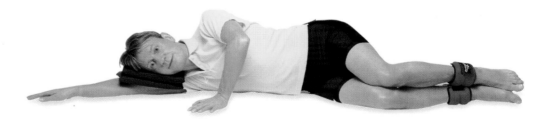

Start position

- Throughout the exercise, keep lifting the waist off the floor and maintain the length in the trunk.
- If you are lucky enough to lack any natural padding around your hip, you may find it uncomfortable to lie like this. If so, just put a small piece of foam underneath your hip.

Action

1. Zipping up and hollowing (stay zipped throughout), take your top leg back, straightening it so that it is in a line with your hip – about twelve centimetres off the floor. Be careful not to take it behind you! Rotate the leg inwards slightly from the hip. The pelvis stays still. Flex the foot towards your face.
2. Breathe out as you slowly lift the leg about fifteen centimetres, then breathe in and lower.
3. Raise and lower the leg ten times, without returning it to the floor. You are breathing out as you raise, in as you lower.
4. Bend the leg to rest on the bent one underneath.
5. Repeat on the other side once you have finished all the other leg-weight exercises on this side.

Watchpoints

- Keep zipping up and hollowing so that you protect the low back and prevent it from arching or the waist dropping down to the floor.
- Lengthen the heel as far away as possible from the hip . . . a long, long, leg, please!
- Keep the rotation inward from the hip, be careful not to turn it in just from the ankle.
- Keep lifting the waist off the floor and lengthening in the body . . . long, long waist.
- Your pelvis should remain absolutely still, do not allow it to roll forward or rock around.
- Don't forget to keep the upper body open, shoulder blades down into your back. Do not allow yourself to roll forward.

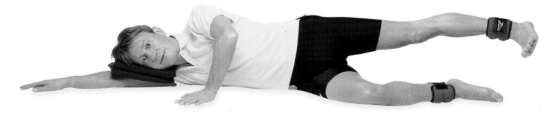

Full position

Twenty Lifts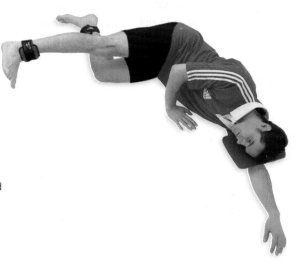

This is a more advanced version of the above, and one which requires a very strong centre.

Aim

To work the gluteals, especially gluteus medius.

Equipment

As for Abductor Lifts.

Action

1. Follow the directions for Abductor Lifts, but this time bring the top straight leg in front of you. Aim to have the leg extended at right angles to you (work up to this).
2. Now raise and lower the leg twenty times, keeping it at hip height and moving it about twelve centimetres up and down, zipping up and hollowing all the time. Breathe normally throughout.

3. After twenty lifts bend the knee back onto the lower leg and give your buttocks a well-earned massage!
4. Repeat on the other side once you have finished all the other leg-weight exercises on this side.

Adductor Lifts

Aim

To tone the inner adductor muscles. To learn pelvic stability.

Equipment

As for Abductor Lifts.

Starting Position

• Lie on your left side as for Abductor Lifts, but now bend your top knee and rest it on a large pillow. The idea is for your pelvis to stay square and not drop forward.

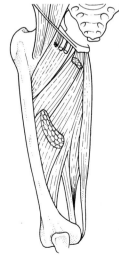

The muscles of the inner thigh – the adductors

- Stretch the bottom leg away a little in front of you, turning it out from the hip joint. Point or flex the foot, either is fine.

Action

1. Breathe in wide and full to prepare.
2. Keeping the leg turned out from the hip, long and straight, breathe out and zip up and hollow (stay zipped now), as you raise the underneath leg slowly. Keep lengthening it away. Do not allow your waist to sink into the floor, keep working it.
3. Breathe in as you lower the leg.
4. Repeat up to twenty times on each side.

Watchpoints

- Keep zipping up and hollowing throughout.
- Don't let the waist sag – keep lengthening it.
- Check that you are moving the whole leg together and not just twisting from the knee.
- Don't let your foot sickle (curl) round to help you come up further. The action must be in the inside of the thigh.
- Check that your upper body stays open, shoulder blades down. Do not roll forward.

When you have completed all the leg-weight exercises, you can then do the complete leg-weight series on the other side.

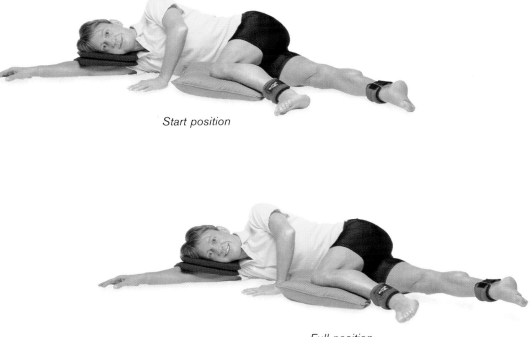

Start position

Full position

Hamstring Scrunches

Aim

To strengthen the hamstrings and buttocks. To stretch the quadriceps.

Equipment

Leg weights.

Starting Position

- Lie on your front.
- Rest your head on your folded hands.
- When you first try this exercise, you may find that you are more comfortable with a pillow under your abdomen.

Action

1. Breathe in wide and full to prepare.
2. Breathe out, zip up and hollow, stay zipped and fold one knee in, bringing the foot towards your bottom. Make sure that as you do so, both hip bones remain on the mat and your lower abdominals stay hollow. Allow the muscles at the front of your thighs to release and lengthen.
3. Breathe in and lower the leg.
4. Repeat up to ten times on each leg.

Watchpoints

- Do not rock from side to side, keep your hip bones firmly on the mat.
- Keep your upper body relaxed.

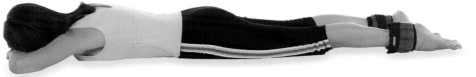

Start position

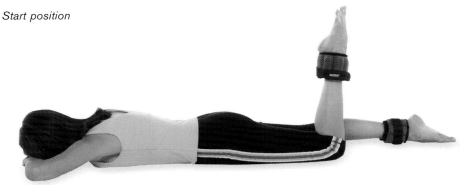

Full position

STRETCHES

Two of these exercises have been described earlier:

Lying Hamstring Stretch see page 58   **Side-lying Quadriceps Stretch see page 56**

Adductor Stretch

Aim

To gently stretch the inner thighs and spine. To focus on lateral lower ribcage breathing.

The wider you place your legs the greater the stretch. This will depend on the flexibility of your hips and the length. Please do not over-stretch.

Starting Position

- Sit on your sitting bones (ischia) with your legs in front of you. If you like you may sit on a rolled up-towel as it will help you to keep your pelvis at the right angle. You could also try sitting with your buttocks against the wall.
- Now take your legs a comfortable distance apart but do not force the knees down into the floor; they may remain a little bent if necessary.
- Have your toes softly pointed until you are very flexible, when you can then have your feet flexed.

Action

1. Breathe in to prepare and lift up out of the hips and lengthen up through the spine. Imagine that there is a pole behind you along your spine, lengthen up along the pole.

2. Breathe out, zip up and hollow and drop your chin forward, gently tucking the chin in. Then, like a roller blind, curl downwards, aiming the top of your head towards the centre of your stomach. Reach forward with your hands.

3. Continue to breathe normally, maintaining navel to spine, and inch forwards reaching through the fingers. If you are flexible enough try to press the knees into the floor, lengthening through the heels.

4. After eight breaths, zipped up and hollowed still, slowly start to unfurl, re-stacking the vertebrae one on top of the other until the spinal column is rebuilt along the length of the imaginary pole. Bring your head up last of all.

5. Repeat three times.

Watchpoints

- Keep your shoulders down into your back, your neck long and released.
- Keep breathing into the back of your ribcage.

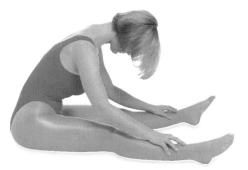

Side Reach and Side Stretch

Aim

To work and stretch your sides!

A lovely exercise which gives you a sense of length and strength throughout your body.

Please take advice if you have low back problems, especially around the sacro-iliac joints at the back of your pelvis.

Equipment

Firm pillow (optional).

Starting Position

- Lie on your side, your underneath leg bent, the thigh at an angle of about 70° to the torso, the lower leg in line with the torso. Your head should similarly be in line with the spine and the underneath arm stretched out in line with the torso (if this is uncomfortable, stretch the arm out at a right angle to the torso and use a thick head support).

- Line up shoulder over shoulder, hip over hip. The 'working leg' should be lined up with the torso and remain parallel and straight with the foot flexed.

- The upper arm lengthens along the body, palm resting on top of the thigh.

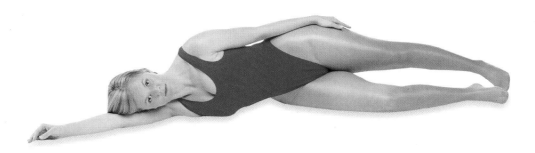

Start position

Action

1. Breathe in wide and full to prepare, the top leg stays straight with the foot on the floor — lengthen away through the heel out of the hip.

2. Breathe out, zip up and hollow, stay zipped now throughout and lift the top leg in parallel just above hip level. At the same time bend from the waist, reaching with the arm towards the knee, sliding the hand along the leg. Eventually, as part of the movement of the torso, your head comes off the mat. Keep your head, neck and spine in good alignment throughout.

3. Breathe in and lift your top arm to touch the floor above you in a line with your body, gently rotating the arm so that the palm faces downward. At the same time, lower the top leg to the floor, lengthening through the heel. Enjoy the stretch.

4. Breathe out, still zipped, and raise the arm and leg simultaneously to repeat action 2 above.

5. Repeat up to five times each side.

Watchpoints

*   Keep the top leg in parallel, do not turn it in or out.
*   Focus straight ahead and maintain the correct alignment of trunk and head. Everything stays in neutral and in line.
*   Keep lengthening your waist.
*   On the stretch part of the exercise think long.

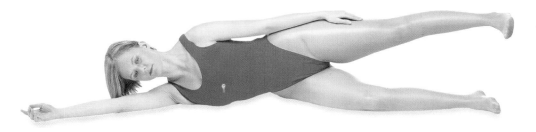

Full position, then take the arm over your head and top foot down to the floor to complete the stretch!

Wind-down

Arm Openings 🚴 🤸

Aim

To open the upper body and stretch the pectoral muscles while stabilising the shoulder blades. To achieve a sense of openness while stabilising and centring. To rotate the spine gently and safely.

As this exercise involves rotation of the spine, please take advice if you have a disc-related injury.

This has to be the most relaxing feel-good exercise in the Pilates programme. Stay completely aware of your arm and hand as it displaces the air moving through space.

Equipment

A pillow and a tennis ball (optional).

Starting Position

- Lie on your side, your head on a pillow, knees curled up at a right angle to your body.
- Your back should be in a 'straight' line, but with its natural curve.
- Place a tennis ball between the knees – the idea is that the tennis ball keeps your knees and pelvis in good alignment.
- Line up all your bones on top of each other – toes, ankles, knees, hips and shoulders.
- Your arms are extended in front of you, palms together at shoulder height.

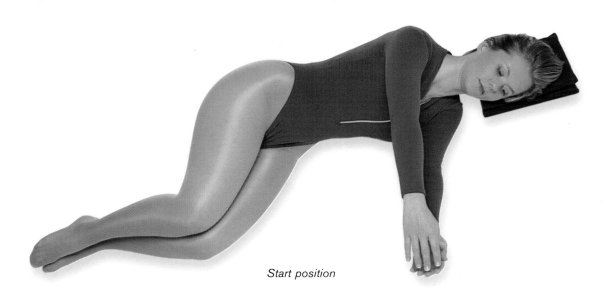

Start position

Action

1. Breathe in to prepare and lengthen through the spine.
2. Breathe out and zip up and hollow.
3. Breathe in as you slowly extend and lift the upper arm, keeping the elbow soft and the shoulder blade down into the back. Keep your eyes on your hand so that the head follows the arm movement. You are aiming to touch the floor behind you, but do not force it. Try to keep your knees together, your pelvis still. Stay zipped up and hollowed.
4. Breathe out as you bring the arm back in an arc to rest on the other hand again.
5. Repeat five times, then curl up on the other side and start again.

Watchpoints

- Keep hollowing throughout.
- Keep your waist long, don't allow it to sink into the floor.
- Don't forget to allow your head to roll naturally with the movement, make sure that it is supported by the pillow.
- Keep the gap between your ears and your shoulders by engaging the muscles below the shoulder blades.

Full position

Relaxation

At last! The perfect way to end the day or the session. Ideally you should persuade a friend to read the instructions to you. Otherwise, try taping them.

Lie in the Relaxation Position, page 24.

- Allow your whole body to melt down into the floor.
- Allow your body to widen and lengthen.
- Take your awareness down to your feet.
- Soften the balls of the feet, uncurling the toes.
- Soften your ankles.
- Soften your calves.
- Release your knees.
- Release your thighs.
- Allow your hips to open.
- Allow the small of your back to sink into the floor as though you are sinking down into the folds of a hammock.
- Feel the length of your spine.
- Take your awareness down to your hands, stretch your fingers away from your palms, feel the centre of your palms opening.
- Then allow the fingers to curl, the palms to soften.
- Allow your elbows to open . . .
- . . . the front of your shoulders to soften.
- With each out-breath, allow your shoulder blades to widen . . .
- . . . your breastbone to soften.

- Allow your neck to release.
- Check your jaw, it should be loose and free.
- Allow your tongue to widen at its base and rest comfortably at the bottom of your mouth.
- Your lips are softly closed.
- Your eyes are softly closed.
- Your forehead is wide and smooth and completely free of lines.
- Your face feels soft.
- Your body is soft and warm.
- Your spine is gently released down into the floor.
- Observe your breathing but do not interrupt it.
- Simply enjoy its natural rhythm . . .

To come out of the Relaxation

- Very gently allow your head to roll to one side, just allow the weight of the head to move it.
- Slowly bring it back to the centre and allow it to roll to the other side . . . bring it back to the centre again.
- Then wiggle your fingers.
- And then, your toes.
- Very slowly roll onto one side and rest there for a few minutes before slowly getting up.

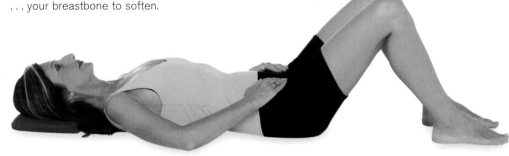

The Relaxation Position

Home Workouts

Workout One

Warm-up

Shoulder Drops	p. 125	
Neck Rolls/Chin Tucks	p. 27	
Spine Curls	p. 58	
Hip Flexor Stretch	p. 105	
Side Rolls	p. 104	
Knee Stirs	p. 126	

Aerobic Warm-up

Now spend five minutes warming up with a gentle aerobic exercise to gently raise your heart rate and body temperature. Choose from:

    Stair climbing

    Skipping

    Walking briskly round the block

    Cycling

Main Workout Including Weights and Stretches

Roll Downs	p. 45	
The Starfish	p. 40	
Curl Ups with Leg Extension	p. 135	
Oblique Curl Ups	p. 99	

The Pelvic Bridge	p. 128	
Flies	p. 144	
Backstroke Swimming	p. 142	
Triceps	p.146	
Biceps	p. 145	
Triceps Stretch	p. 93	
Abductor Lifts	p. 150	
Adductor Lifts	p. 152	
Side Reach and Side Stretch	p. 156	
Lying Hamstring Stretch	p. 106	
Standing Quadriceps Stretch	p. 54	
The Dart Stage Two	p. 110	
Rest Position	p. 109	

Wind-down

Arm Openings	p. 158	
Relaxation	p. 160	

Workout Two

Warm-up

Shoulder Drops	p. 125	
Neck Rolls/Chin Tucks	p. 27	
Spine Curls	p. 106	
Hip Flexor Stretch	p. 105	
Side Rolls	p. 104	
Knee Stirs	p. 126	

Aerobic Warm-up

Now spend five minutes warming up with a gentle aerobic exercise to gently raise your heart rate and body temperature. Choose from:

Stair climbing

Skipping

Walking briskly round the block

Cycling

Main Workout Including Weights and Stretches

The Starfish	p. 40	
Pelvic Stability Check	p. 34	
Arm Openings	p. 158	
Curl Ups with Leg Extension	p. 135	
Windows	p. 129	

Roll Downs	p. 46	
The Corkscrew	p. 49	
Waist Twists	p. 51	
Walking on the Spot	p. 52	
Back Scrub	p. 133	
Reverse Dips	p. 134	
Triceps Stretch	p. 93	
Hamstring Scrunches	p. 154	
Lying Hamstring Stretch	p. 58	
Side-lying Quadriceps Stretch	p. 56	
Push-ups	p. 138, 139, 140	
Diamond Press	p. 136	
Rest Position	p. 109	
Single Leg Stretch	p. 100	

Wind-down

Pillow Squeeze	p. 110	
Relaxation	p. 160	

Workout Three

Warm-up

Shoulder Drops	p. 125	
Neck Rolls/Chin Tucks	p. 27	
Spine Curls	p. 106	
Hip Flexor Stretch	p. 105	
Side Rolls	p. 104	
Knee Stirs	p. 126	

Aerobic Warm-up

Now spend five minutes warming up with a gentle aerobic exercise to gently raise your heart rate and body temperature. Choose from:

Stair climbing

Skipping

Walking briskly round the block

Cycling

Main Workout Including Weights and Stretches

The Starfish	p. 40	
Pelvic Stability – Knee Turnout	p. 36	
Pillow Squeeze	p. 110	
Windows	p. 129	
Waist Twists	p. 51	

Walking on the Spot	p. 52	
Standing Quadriceps Stretch	p. 54	
Pec Stretch: Through the Doorway	p. 87	
The Dart Stage Two	p. 108	
Rest Position	p. 109	
Curl Ups with Leg Extension	p. 135	
Single Leg Stretch	p. 100	
Arm Openings	p. 158	
Side Reach and Side Stretch	p. 156	
Lying Hamstring Stretch	p. 58	
Wall Stretch One	p. 148	
Wall Stretch Two	p. 149	

Wind-down

Roll Downs Against a Wall	p. 130	
Relaxation	p. 160	

Workout Four

Warm-up

Shoulder Drops	p. 125	
Neck Rolls/Chin Tucks	p. 27	
Spine Curls	p. 106	
Hip Flexor Stretch	p. 105	
Side Rolls	p. 104	
Knee Stirs	p. 126	

Aerobic warm-up

Now spend five minutes warming up with a gentle aerobic exercise to gently raise your heart rate and body temperature. Choose from:

    Stair climbing

    Skipping

    Walking briskly round the block

    Cycling

Main Workout Including Weights and Stretches

The Starfish	p. 40	
Pillow Squeeze	p. 110	
Roll Downs	p. 46	
The Corkscrew	p. 49	
Waist Twists	p. 51	

Back Scrub	p. 133	
Hamstring Scrunches	p. 154	
Lying Hamstring Stretch	p. 58	
Side-lying Quadriceps Stretch	p. 56	
Adductor Stretch	p. 155	
Single Leg Stretch	p. 100	
Push-ups (non-machine) – two to three sets, eight to twelve repetitions	p. 138, 139, 140	
Diamond Press	p. 136	
Rest Position	p. 109	

Wind-down

Arm Openings	p. 158	
Relaxation	p. 160	

Workout Five

Warm-up

Shoulder Drops	p. 125	
Neck Rolls/Chin Tucks	p. 27	
Spine Curls	p. 106	
Hip Flexor Stretch	p. 105	
Side Rolls	p. 104	
Knee Stirs	p. 126	

Aerobic Warm-up

Now spend five minutes warming up with a gentle aerobic exercise to gently raise your heart rate and body temperature. Choose from:

Stair climbing

Skipping

Walking briskly round the block

Cycling

Main Workout Including Weights and Stretches

The Starfish	p. 40	
Pelvic Stability Check	p. 34	
Arm Openings	p. 158	
Curl Ups with Leg Extension	p. 135	
Roll Downs Against the Wall	p. 130	

Shoulder Circles	p. 48	
Neck Crescents	p. 50	
Pec Stretch: Through the Doorway	p. 87	
Flies	p. 144	
Backstroke Swimming	p. 142	
Triceps	p. 146	
Biceps	p. 145	
Wall Stretch One	p. 148	
Wall Stretch Two	p. 149	
Abductor Lifts	p. 150	
Adductor Lifts	p. 152	
Side Reach and Side Stretch	p. 156	
Adductor Stretch	p. 155	
Lying Hamstring Stretch	p. 58	
The Dart Stage Two	p. 108	
Rest Position	p. 109	

Wind-down

Relaxation	p. 160	

Workout Six

Warm-up

Shoulder Drops	p. 125	
Neck Rolls/Chin Tucks	p. 27	
Spine Curls	p. 106	
Hip Flexor Stretch	p. 105	
Side Rolls	p. 104	
Knee Stirs	p. 126	

Aerobic Warm-up

Now spend five minutes warming up with a gentle aerobic exercise to gently raise your heart rate and body temperature. Choose from:

> Stair climbing
> Skipping
> Walking briskly round the block
> Cycling

Main Workout Including Weights and Stretches

Shoulder Circles	p. 48	
Neck Crescents	p. 50	
Waist Twists	p. 51	
Roll Downs	p. 46	
Back Scrub	p. 133	

Windows	p. 129	
Curl Ups with Leg Extension	p. 135	
Oblique Curl Ups	p. 99	
Diamond Press	p. 136	
Rest Position	p. 109	
Hamstrings Scrunches	p. 154	
Reverse Dips	p. 134	
Side Reach and Side Stretch	p. 156	
Lying Hamstring Stretch	p. 58	
Single Leg Stretch	p. 100	

Wind-down

Arm Openings	p. 158	
Pillow Squeeze	p. 110	
Relaxation	p. 160	

Workout Seven

Warm-up

Shoulder Drops	p. 125	
Neck Rolls/Chin Tucks	p. 27	
Spine Curls	p. 106	
Hip Flexor Stretch	p. 105	
Side Rolls	p. 104	
Knee Stirs	p. 126	

Aerobic warm-up

Now spend five minutes warming up with a gentle aerobic exercise to gently raise your heart rate and body temperature. Choose from:

- Stair climbing
- Skipping
- Walking briskly round the block
- Cycling

Main Workout Including Weights and Stretches

Shoulder Circles	p. 48	
Neck Crescents	p. 50	
Roll Downs	p. 46	
The Corkscrew	p. 49	
The Pelvic Bridge	p. 128	

Curl Ups with Leg Extension	p. 135	
Oblique Curl Ups	p. 99	
Flies	p. 144	
Backstroke Swimming	p. 142	
Triceps	p. 146	
Biceps	p. 145	
Wall Stretch One	p. 148	
Wall Stretch Two	p. 149	
Abductor Lifts	p. 150	
Adductor Lifts	p. 152	
Adductor Stretch	p. 155	
Lying Hamstring Stretch	p. 58	
Side Reach and Side Stretch	p. 156	
Diamond Press	p. 136	
Rest Position	p. 109	

Wind-down

Relaxation	p. 160	

Further Information

For more information on Body Control Pilates,
please visit *www.bodycontrol.co.uk*

or contact

Body Control Pilates USA
Eastside Studio
Suite 110
3100 Richmond Street
Houston
TX 77098

Balanced Body Inc
7500 14th Avenue
Suite 23
Sacramento
CA 95820-3539
www.balancedbody.com

Video
Lynne Robinson's videos 'Body Control' (WSP241)
and 'Weekly Workout'
(WSP242)
are available from good video stores or from
Wellspring Media at
www.wellmedia.com

Background Reading

On Pilates

Body Control: The Pilates Way, Lynne Robinson and Gordon Thomson, Boxtree, 1997

The Body Control Pilates Manual, Lynne Robinson, Helge Fisher, Jacqueline Knox, Gordon Thomson, Pan Books, 2000

Every Body is Beautiful, Ron Fletcher, Lippencott, 1978 (out of print)

How to Improve Your Posture, Fran Lehen, Cornerstone Library, 1982

The Mind Body Workout, Lynne Robinson and Helge Fisher, Pan Books, 1998

Pilates The Way Forward, Lynne Robinson and Gordon Thomson, Pan Books,1999

The Pilates Method of Physical and Mental Conditioning, Philip Friedman and Gail Eisen, Warner Books, 1980

General

'Dysfunction of Tranversus Abdominus associated with Chronic Low Back Pain', article by P. W. Hodges, Department of Physiotherapy, The University of Queensland, *MPAA Conference Proceedings*, 1995

'Muscle Control – Pain Control. What exercises would you prescribe?', article by C. A. Richardson and G. A. Jull, Department of Physiotherapy, University of Queensland, Australia, *Manual Therapy*, Pearson Professional Ltd., 1995

Anatomy of Movement, Blandine Calais-Germain, Eastland Press, 1993

Body Fitness and Exercise – Basic Theory and Practice for Therapists, Mo Rosser, Hodder and Stoughton, 1995

Body Stories – A Guide To Experiential Anatomy, Andrea Olsen, Station Hill Press, 1991

Dance Kinesiology, Sally Sevey Fitt, Schirmer, 1988

Dancing Longer, Dancing Stronger, Andrea Watkins and Priscilla M. Clarkson, Princeton Book Company, 1990

Flexibility, Principles and Practice, Christopher Norris, Black, 1994

Human Movement Potential – Its Ideokinetic Facilitation, Lulu Swiegard, Harper and Row Publishers Inc., University Press of America Inc., 1974

Manual of Structural Kinesiology, Clem Thompson, Times Mirror/Mosby College Publishing, 1989

Muscle Testing and Function, Kendall, Kendall and Wadsworth, Williams and Wilkins, Baltimore/ London, 1971

Sports Injuries – Diagnosis and Management for Physiotherapists, Christopher Norris, Butterworth Heinemann, 1993

The Anatomy Coloring Book, Wynn Kapit and Lawrence M. Elson, HarperCollins, 1977

The Art Of Changing – A New Approach to the Alexander Technique, Glen Park, Ashgrove Press Ltd., 1989

The Body Has Its Reasons: Anti-Exercises and Self-Awareness, Therese Bertherat and Carol Bernstein, Cedar, 1988

Therapeutic Exercise Foundations and Techniques, Carolyn Kisner and Lynn Allen Colby, F. A. Davis Company, 1990

Your Body, Biofeedback at its Best, B. J. Jencks, Nelson Hall, Chicago, 1977